"The new mind-body manual." —Style.com

"*Eat Pretty* is a must-read for every woman who wants to glow." —Sophie Uliano, *New York Times* bestselling author of *Gorgeously Green*

"That beautiful glow you get from your green smoothies? *Eat Pretty* has it down to a science. This book has everything you need to boost the pretty in your plant-based diet." —Kris Carr, *New York Times* bestselling author of *Crazy Sexy Kitchen*

"*Eat Pretty* reveals the secrets of true beauty from the inside out. Beauty-full reading to last a lifetime." —Ann Louise Gittleman, PhD, CNS, *New York Times* bestselling author of *The Fat Flush Plan* and *The Living Beauty Detox Program*

EAT PRETTY

NUTRITION for BEAUTY,
INSIDE and OUT

Jolene Hart, CHC, AADP

CHRONICLE BOOKS

SAN FRANCISCO

To my mom, who taught me that food is medicine,
and my dad, who showed me that laughter is, too.
And to Rob, who makes every day more beautiful.

Text copyright © 2014 by Jolene Hart.
Illustrations copyright © 2014 by Chronicle Books LLC.
All rights reserved. No part of this book may be reproduced in any form without written permission from the publisher.

Library of Congress Cataloging-in-Publication Data:
Hart, Jolene.
  Eat pretty / by Jolene Hart.
    pages cm
  Includes index.
  ISBN 978-1-4521-2366-0 (alk. paper)
  1. Nutrition. 2. Beauty, Personal. 3. Functional foods. I. Title.
  RA784.H369 2014
  613.2—dc23

                    2013026812

Manufactured in China

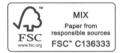

Designed by Allison Weiner
Illustrations by Vikki Chu
Typesetting by Frank Brayton

The opinions expressed in this book are solely those of Jolene Hart, a health coach certified by the Institute for Integrative Nutrition and the American Association of Drugless Practitioners, who does not dispense medical advice and is not acting in the capacity of a licensed physician, dietician, nutritionist, psychologist, or other licensed or registered professional. The information presented in this book should not be construed as medical advice and is not meant to replace treatment by licensed health-care professionals. Please consult your physcian or professional health-care advisor regarding your specific health-care needs before making any changes to your diet, lifestyle, or medical treatment regimen. Use of the information in this book is at the reader's own discretion and risk. The author and Chronicle Books hereby disclaim any and all liability resulting from injuries, loss, or damage caused by following any recommendations contained in this book.

20 19 18 17 16 15 14

Chronicle Books LLC
680 Second Street
San Francisco, California 94107
www.chroniclebooks.com

CONTENTS

FIND YOUR HEALTHY VANITY

Imagine you're a beauty editor at a major magazine. You have access to all the makeup, styling products, nail polish, cutting-edge skin care and perfumes you can handle, and you get them all before your friends and family. Did I mention that they don't cost you a thing, because it's your *job* to test them? You can call up any beauty company and they'll gladly rush you the product that you're coveting, and half a dozen others. You also get facials, blowouts, haircuts, massages, manicures (performed at your desk, if necessary), pedicures, and the like pretty regularly; all in a day's work. Some would say you have it all. All except the one thing you want most: clear skin.

Welcome to my personal nightmare.

My painfully irritated complexion was just one sign that I was coming up short on healthy beauty tools. There was the itchy eczema on my legs, the dark circles under my eyes, the expanding waistline—but that wasn't even the extent of it. I didn't *feel* beautiful either. I didn't have energy or sparkle the way I knew I should. When I realized that I had just about every beauty product in existence at my fingertips and yet I wasn't a step closer to looking and feeling my best, I started searching for an answer beyond the beauty aisle. I needed real solutions, and the conventional lineup of treatments, products, and prescriptions had already failed. Where was that magic product that would restore the beauty and well-being that was my birthright?

If you've been asking yourself the same question, I welcome you into this space. You, along with millions of other women around the world, are ready for a powerful new approach to your beauty: Eat Pretty. The information in this book brought beauty back into my life, cleared my skin, rebuilt my relationship with food, helped me become more resilient to the effects of stress, and enabled me to create a lifestyle of beauty that supports my body and mind every day. My Eat Pretty journey was a more pampering, empowering, and transformative experience than I ever imagined it would be. You too have a transformation ahead of you, one that requires you to look beyond quick fixes. Looking and feeling your best means exploring good digestion, healthy hormones, restful sleep, emotional health and, as the foundation of it all, Eat Pretty foods that support your beauty and wellness. Each of these beauty players contributes to your ultimate goal: to reveal your most radiant self. I'll discuss their functions in detail in the pages ahead.

You may already know that good nutrition is more than just getting your recommended daily allowance of vitamins and minerals, or adhering to a "calories in, calories out" equation. You may have adopted diets designed to help with issues from weight loss to allergies to mood. But so many of us possess a foundational understanding of nutrition without an appreciation of the deep connection between food and beauty. It's time to learn one vital nutritional lesson: that the power to shape all aspects of our appearance, today and in the future, lies on our plates. One can have an underlying knowledge of good health and nutrition, as I did, and still fail to create a diet and lifestyle that supports beauty. So many of the foods readily available to us today are sneaky saboteurs of our looks that tempt us with promises of weight loss, convenience, or adventurous eating. I filled my diet with them, unknowingly. I also didn't take time to cook meals from whole, unprocessed foods, or even establish a regular mealtime. I saw food as an enemy, a vice, or a cover for my emotions. And I listened to advice from experts who assured me that there was no connection between my skin problems and my diet, even though I sensed that my blemishes and rashes were cries for help from my body. But all of that changed when I learned to eat for beauty.

In this age of unprecedented exploration in nutritional science, the groundbreaking research and mind-blowing discoveries happening around us finally prove something about beauty that is as familiar as it is true, simple, and fundamental: we are what we eat. I can hear the groans already. *"Ugh, I guess I'm a Diet Coke, a grilled cheese sandwich, and a side of fries."* Or, *"Well, I look pretty good, but I don't feel great . . . am I all those years of microwave popcorn and Cosmopolitans?"* But I say, "Absolutely not!" Even if your eating habits were less than beautiful yesterday, boosting your beauty nutrition will have a major impact on your glow and energy *today*. Once I freed my own diet from processed snacks, diet sodas, and inflammation-causing foods and replaced them with fresh, living beauty foods, the longstanding burden was lifted from my body and skin.

This news is incredibly empowering—*we write our beauty story with every bite*—so don't feel overwhelmed at the changes that you may want to make as you work your way through this book. I promise, the Eat Pretty lifestyle feels so true to *you* that you won't crave anything less for your beautiful life. Get excited that you have a hand in your beauty. Actually, you have two hands—one for your fork and one for your knife.

I created the Eat Pretty program to be the perfect complement to your current beauty routine; it's a lifestyle that will deepen your beauty many times over, giving you a stunning canvas for the products you already love. In this compact volume built to accompany you through your busy and fabulous life, *Eat Pretty* explains in detail exactly how to put your beautifying lifestyle into practice. We'll concentrate on the factors you strongly influence, to start you on the path to gorgeous for life.

My approach to beauty borrows from my experience as a beauty editor and journalist, my personal search for beauty and wellness, and my work as a health coach. In Part 1 of this book, Rethink Beauty, I explain why a one-sided beauty routine limits your glow, and how the wrong food choices could be sabotaging your beauty from within. In Part 2, Four Seasons to Eat Pretty, you'll learn about more than eighty-five foods that deepen your beauty from the inside out. Part 3, The Essential Beauty Players, reveals that diet is by no means the only influencer of healthy beauty. Stress, digestion, environment, sleep, emotions, and yes, genetics, all factor into the beauty equation. My goal in writing *Eat Pretty* was to unite what we know about many different areas of health to create your new beauty toolkit.

You'll find that I take the middle road in my beautifying lifestyle: I devour every tidbit of science related to nutrition, aging, and healthy beauty, but I'm also influenced by the traditional wisdom surrounding beauty (like why we just seem to look more radiant when we're happier!) that's tricky to document using scientific methods. So the principles of

Eat Pretty mix the teachings of Eastern traditions with modern nutritional science, genetic research, and the most up-to-date dermatological findings. Unlike hundreds of the beauty products you might buy over a lifetime, *Eat Pretty* is one tool that will change your relationship with beauty by changing the way you understand your body.

My beauty story is just one of countless others like it. If you've ever wanted to change your skin, your weight, your hair, or just about anything else about yourself, you know how powerfully your looks influence your sense of self. Changing your looks really can change your life. Our appearance shapes the way we feel about ourselves—and that reflects in our confidence, in our decision-making, in our overall joy, even in the way we treat others. Eating for beauty has a similar snowball effect. Start with small changes in your meals and you set in motion a momentum that shifts the way you feel and the way you look, which in turn influences your posture, your grooming habits, your actions, and so many of your choices.

The Eat Pretty lifestyle will remake your relationship with food and change your understanding of your beauty and body. At the same time, you'll build an antiaging lifestyle that supports you today, not to mention when you're forty, fifty, sixty, and beyond. Just what force inspires us to make these changes, and to better our beauty and body? To me it's a universal quality that I call "healthy vanity"—although there's nothing vain about it. Healthy vanity is our desire to look and feel our best, and to show that best self to the world. It's the beauty we were born to have. Now is your time to own it. As you rethink your approach to beauty and self-care, I want you to keep in mind just how much influence you have over your body. That's what I find most empowering about Eat Pretty, and I hope you will, too.

Whenever you need inspiration to stick to Eat Pretty, just look in the mirror. Let your healthy vanity take over for a moment. We all want to feel beautiful in our own personal ways. But the root of our desires is profoundly similar. We want to love ourselves. We want to be loved. And we want our outer beauty to reflect the incredible being we are inside. You are ready to look your best, not for a day or a week, but for life. To achieve this you need the right tools. Think of the potted plant on your windowsill. You forget to water it and it wilts. Starve it of light and it grows weak and spindly reaching for the sun. Deny it adequate nutrients and it develops spots, wrinkles, brown leaves, and its color fades. It ages prematurely. Without these forms of essential nourishment, you can expect a plant that's just barely getting by, one that might not have the energy to produce flowers or fruit this season.

When it comes to your own appearance, the rule stands: skimp on essential beauty nutrition, and your beauty simply can't flourish. It's not to say that your beauty isn't there—it's just missing the right components. You may have already noticed that your skin, hair, and nails are often the first parts of your body to expose an internal imbalance. Dull, dry, blemished skin, damaged hair, and weight gain signal that something is amiss inside—and diet and lifestyle are the first places to look to restore your radiant glow. The good news is that your beauty, like the plants that perk up when revived with water and sunlight and grow back season after season, is resilient. You never have to settle for wilted blossoms. Nourish your beauty from the inside and watch yourself bloom. The results will speak for themselves, every time you look in the mirror or walk into a room.

While writing this book, I heard from so many women that they loved the title. *Eat Pretty*. Two crisp, neat little words; a perfect package. If only beauty were so clearly defined. Your embodiment of beauty may be different from your neighbor's, but the same steps to nourishing beauty apply to us all. The confidence achieved by looking and feeling your best and showing that radiant self to the world is the "pretty" that we all desire. And it's yours for the taking when you support your beauty from the inside. Your gorgeous future begins with your very next meal. Beauty isn't manifest destiny; it's a journey guided by your daily choices. If you're ready to choose radiance, energy, glow, youth, and vitality, follow me to the Eat Pretty life.

Let's turn beauty inside out.

In beauty and health,

Jolene

At one time or another, we've all been taught that our dietary choices influence our health outcomes. But for far too long we've given little to no regard to the fact that our beauty—the way we look and feel and move through every moment of our lives—is a direct reflection of that state of health. Beauty is wellness. Wellness is beauty. This is the essence of *Eat Pretty*.

So, what should and shouldn't you expect from this unique beauty guide? As we work together to shape your personal lifestyle of beauty, keep in mind:

- There are no overnight miracles (you won't find them in foods *or* beauty products). If you expect to wake up with hair that has grown silky-smooth overnight after eating half of a butternut squash, you'll miss the point of *Eat Pretty*—and be sorely disappointed by the lack of results. Instead, think of it like this: Every bite is an opportunity to boost your outer glow, deeply and over time.
- Not all foods are created equal. Some may have documented nutritional benefits and appear to be fine for all diets but still may be common triggers for beauty concerns. For this reason, you'll find very little, if any, gluten, dairy, refined sugar, or meat in your beauty diet.
- *Eat Pretty* shapes your approach to food and lifestyle, but achieving optimal beauty is also about listening to your own unique body and understanding how it responds to all forms of nourishment. You'll always be prettiest when you eat what's right for *you*.
- It's not radical news that pumpkin seeds are a terrific source of zinc, or that strawberries are packed with vitamin C. But it *is* groundbreaking to apply this nutritional know-how to your existing beauty routine. Learn to see foods in a different way— as friends, not foes—and recognize that beauty is a sign of health that blossoms from within.

PART 1

RETHINK BEAUTY

*Y*ou're about to undergo a stunning transformation that begins with rethinking beauty. With *Eat Pretty* in hand, you've made the choice to show up for life bright-eyed, energetic, vibrant, glowing, and healthy. You no longer want to see beauty and feel beautiful only when under a cover of foundation and lipstick. You want your best self in every breath, thought, step, and yes, every bite. And you're ready to create your unique lifestyle of beauty from within. In the next three chapters, I'll help you identify the foods, habits, and thoughts that have been holding you back from your most beautiful life, and teach you the basic ways to nourish radiance from the inside. Radiant beauty is your best accessory. It beats the "it" bag, the shoe of the moment, and the most coveted pair of jeans. It's a symbol of glamour and style, but it doesn't take big bucks to get it. It's accessible to *all* women. When you let the Eat Pretty lifestyle guide you, pampering you with the most beautifying foods and habits at every turn, you'll never see your beauty the same way again.

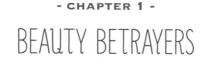

- CHAPTER 1 -

BEAUTY BETRAYERS

From the moment your soles hit the floor in the morning, your beauty endures an endless stream of assaults from the outside. Your skin, hair, and nails get hit from every angle: UV rays from the sun, environmental pollution in the air, toxins in your products, stress at the office—not to mention regular scrubbing, tanning, brushing, blow-drying . . . you get the picture. To avoid these outside beauty stressors completely, you'd have to stay under the covers!

While we can't eliminate outside beauty saboteurs from our daily lives, we can stop ourselves from creating an additional beauty burden *inside* our bodies. This means freeing our diets of what I call Beauty Betrayers: the foods that actually do damage to our healthy skin, hair, nails, weight, and moods. Beauty Betrayers may taste great and seem harmless when they pass between your lips, but they're just plain lousy for long-term glow. Beauty Betrayers cause inflammation and digestive difficulties, increase your body's toxic load, speed up the aging process, and generally throw a troublesome wrench in your healthy vanity. To add insult to injury, they don't supply the building blocks that your body needs to perform its essential processes of repair, detox, and defense. They leave you feeling exhausted, moody, and craving even more foods that stress your beauty from the inside out. The only way to stop the cycle—and regain your gorgeous glow—is to kick them off your plate. You're about to find out how easy and delicious that can be!

BEAUTY BETRAYER FOODS

Here's where things get ugly. To truly transform your beauty and health, you must first weed out the foods that undermine your beauty. Steer clear of—or seriously limit—the following Beauty Betrayer foods to lift the un-pretty burden from your body and defend against aging before your time.

Alcohol It's fun to raise a glass in celebration, but alcohol does no favors for your beauty. Every time you imbibe, you consume empty calories that offer zero nutritional benefits to your body and actually steal nutrition and hydration from your beauty. Alcohol, like sugar, disrupts delicate hormonal balance. It also stresses your liver—a very important organ for a glowing complexion—and affects blood flow to your skin, leaving you either lackluster or flushed with broken capillaries. If you choose to indulge, remember to do so in moderation to avoid a major beauty hangover!

Caffeine That cup of coffee perks you up temporarily, but it also pumps up the stress hormone cortisol, which contributes to wrinkles and belly fat around your middle, not to mention the jitters! Caffeine puts a major burden on your body's adrenal glands and liver, and it's acidic to your body's pH (see page 54 for more on unhealthy acidity). Drinking caffeine can also prevent you from getting deep, reparative beauty sleep.

Canned Foods with Bisphenol A Studies link it to breast cancer, depression, and childhood obesity, but you might not realize that endocrine-disrupting bisphenol A (BPA), the chemical found in the lining of almost all canned food, is also a downer for your looks. BPA mimics estrogen in your body, throwing off your natural hormonal balance, which is essential for everything from reproduction to clear skin and healthy aging. Skip canned food that's been exposed to BPA and go for fresh foods—or those packed in BPA-free cans.

Dairy Skin looking spotty? You may want to put down that ice cream cone. The average non-organic, or "conventional," dairy products at your grocery store contain antibiotics and added hormones that spike insulin in the body, leading to breakouts. The hormones in conventional dairy are powerful enough to throw off your body's natural hormonal balance (see page 173 for more on hormonal balance). Milk consumption in particular may cause a 10 to 20 percent rise in a key oil-producing hormone in adults that can fuel unwanted acne.

Dairy, both organic and conventional, is also one of the most common food intolerances. Two troubling components of dairy, a protein called casein and a sugar called lactose, can cause bloating and gas, as well as digestive issues that prevent your body from breaking down and assimilating the essential nutrients from your beauty foods. Dairy products are also acidic in the body. For those who do eat dairy, raw or organic products from grass-fed animals are better choices to minimize hormone intake, while goat and sheep cheeses can be more easily digestible than cow's-milk cheese.

Fried Foods It's not just that fried foods are high in fat; they're often loaded with un-pretty fat sources like cooked oils and trans fats. Oils that have been heated to a high temperature for frying purposes become major sources of free radicals, reactive oxygen molecules that steal electrons from healthy molecules in your body, causing cellular damage in the process. Free radicals in fried foods cause wrinkles, inflammation, age spots, and head-to-toe beauty issues! Those harmless-looking fries are also likely to be hidden sources of trans fats, if you live in an area that has yet to ban these harmful hydrogenated compounds. Trans fats have been linked to obesity, inflammation, high cholesterol, and heart disease, and they can aggravate, even cause, a hormonal imbalance in your body.

Gluten You may not realize that even if you don't have celiac disease—a serious gluten allergy—you could still be highly sensitive to gluten, a protein found in many grains including wheat, rye, and barley. Gluten sensitivity is difficult to diagnose, even with a blood test, so we often unknowingly experience gluten's negative effects, such as inflammation that speeds up aging and leads to weight gain; compromised digestion and assimilation of beauty nutrients; and a harmful immune response. If you have persistent skin problems or poor digestion, your relationship with gluten is important to consider. Gluten sensitivity can also manifest itself in headaches, fatigue, and redness and advanced aging of the skin.

Grilled and Overcooked Foods The more you burn, brown, singe, and generally overcook your foods, the less beauty nutrients they retain—and the more wrinkle-causing Advanced Glycation End Products (AGEs) they form in your body when you eat them. As you'll read on page 24, AGEs speed up signs of aging like wrinkles, age spots, and sagging skin, and increase inflammation and weight gain. Charred meats are especially damaging to beauty, since animal proteins are prone to AGE formation and dry, high-temperature grilling methods make things even worse; but charred veggies are also problematic for beauty. Try steaming, sautéing with water or broth, or poaching your foods—quickly is key—to keep AGE formation to a minimum, and do not eat burned food. This isn't to say that you should shut down your barbecue grill for good; just be aware of heat levels and cooking time. And try eating a few more raw, antioxidant-rich foods to neutralize those free radicals!

Meats (Conventional) So much of the meat eaten today, including cryptically named "meat products," come from animals fed antibiotics, hormones, and other un-pretty ingredients. Most "conventional" meats available to you at the supermarket boost inflammation with an abundance of omega-6 fatty acids and a lack of omega-3s (see page 49), the opposite of what you want for beauty and health. Eating meat at every meal, or even several times a week, also crowds out opportunities to eat more beautifying sources of protein. If you do choose to eat animal protein, a better choice is hormone-free, grass-fed meat, in moderation, or wild-caught fish free from high mercury levels. Some types of fish are fantastic sources of omega-3s, which is one of the reasons I recommend them in your Eat Pretty diet. Skip red meat and poultry in favor of other proteins like salmon, spirulina, pastured eggs (from hens that have access to sunlight, outdoor space, and natural protein sources like bugs and worms—they're richer in omega-3s and vitamins A, D, and E), quinoa, and lentils. You'll find that they pack much more beauty bang for your buck.

Pesticide-Sprayed Produce Unless you buy organic produce, you'll likely be exposed to pesticide residue containing toxins that increase the free-radical burden on your body and interfere with other beauty defense and repair processes. Try to eat organic whenever possible; the fewer pesticides and additives that your body has to contend with, the more energy it has to keep you beautiful and protect your organs from accumulating a harmful toxic load. Reducing your intake of pesticides can even help you keep off unwanted weight.

Processed Foods Processed foods created to withstand weeks, months, or years on the shelf are hardly living fuel for your beauty. They contribute preservatives, chemical additives, synthetic dyes, and fake flavors to your diet, but skimp on beautifying ingredients. Processed ingredients trigger aging inflammation and load your body with free radicals. And many processed foods—think baked goods, cereals, chips, candy bars, and crackers—rank high on the glycemic index, meaning that each time you eat them, they cause a spike in blood sugar that contributes to acne, wrinkles, and hormonal imbalance. We're so used to the grab-and-go convenience of processed foods that we forget just how many other un-pretty ingredients they also contain. Swap processed foods, including frozen meals, premade veggie burgers, granola bars, and other packaged snacks, for fresh foods and you free up major energy for your body to rejuvenate, repair, and boost your overall beauty and health.

Soda Liquid calories: what have they done for you lately? One can of soda is highly acidic and contains nearly 10 teaspoons of refined sugar, which places a major aging burden on your body. Diet soda is no better, since it's loaded with artificial sweeteners that can slow your metabolism and cause you to pack on the pounds. High levels of phosphates in soda have been linked to accelerated aging, including skin atrophy (which shows up as thinning, wrinkling skin), tooth enamel decay, and bone loss. Caramel color in colas is a direct source of AGE formation, an aging, wrinkle-causing process.

Sugar Ready to go into sugar shock? Sweet treats made with refined sugar are more than just bad news for your waistline: sugar directly contributes to wrinkles, age spots, blemishes, lackluster skin, and cellulite. Sugar is just plain toxic to your beauty. It's a major cause of AGE formation in the body, which leads to the breakdown of collagen (the main structural protein supporting healthy skin), connective tissue, and even your vascular system. Your sweet tooth may be fun to indulge in the moment, but it's also highly addictive—not to mention acidic and inflammatory in the body. Sugar steals nutrients and hydration from your skin; suppresses your immune system, making you more prone to illness; feeds bad bacteria; and curbs the production of antiaging hormones in your body.

Another reason to watch out for foods with added sugar: eating sugar is likely to block your brain from effectively signaling fullness and satiation, which could cause you to overindulge. And when your body uses energy to process sugar, fat-burning takes a back seat, so skipping refined sugar could rev up your metabolism and weight loss. Artificial sweeteners are not only toxic, they can also cause water retention, bloating, indigestion, headaches, sugar cravings, and weight gain, so unfortunately, they're no more beautiful—or slimming—than other sugars.

Still have a major sweet tooth? Check out my favorite sweeteners on page 71 for a splurge. You'll learn in the pages ahead that eating sugar in moderation and in combination with other blood sugar–steadying foods, like cinnamon, fiber, or protein, can reduce its un-pretty effects.

BEAUTY BETRAYERS: THE UGLY CONSEQUENCES

A diet full of Beauty Betrayers leaves you ill-prepared to fight off the outside attacks on your beauty. But the news gets worse. Each of those harmful foods is enough to cause a beauty breakdown on its own. Even if you don't see blemishes, brittle hair, and dull skin after guzzling down a diet soda, you can be certain that Beauty Betrayer foods are hard at work sabotaging your beauty from the inside, and soon enough there will be visible consequences. Rather than providing abundant antioxidants, enzymes, vitamins, minerals, and amino acids to support your gorgeous glow, Beauty Betrayers steal beauty energy and burden your body with pesticides, synthetic dyes, preservatives, trans fats, and ingredients like caffeine, alcohol, and refined sugar that *promote* aging.

Your diet can speed up aging, or it can serve as your greatest defense. Which do you choose? Eat Pretty foods send protective messages to your body, while Beauty Betrayers send dysfunctional messages that hold back your beauty and health. Beauty, like life, is a series of choices! So what'll it be? Your diet can . . .

- create free radicals, or neutralize them.
- turn on genes for disease, or switch them off.
- leave you more susceptible to sun damage, or protect you from UV rays.
- increase inflammation, or reduce inflammation.
- cause excessive acidity, or promote ideal alkalinity.

- ☒ compromise the healthy bacteria in your digestive system, or support their growth.
- ☒ contribute to oxidative stress levels, or serve as your body's greatest stress defense.
- ☒ form AGEs in your body, or prevent them.
- ☒ damage DNA function, or protect it.

To shed a little more light on the havoc that Beauty Betrayers wreak on an otherwise look-good, feel-good lifestyle, the sections that follow explain the damaging internal processes triggered when the wrong foods get a regular place in your diet. Here's what happens *after* Beauty Betrayer foods hit your lips:

Free Radical Free-for-All Wondering where aging starts? There's an incriminating finger pointing at free radicals, reactive oxygen molecules that are missing an electron. Free radicals form as a result of unprotected exposure to UV rays, pollution, pesticides, cigarette smoke, and radiation, as well as from oxidized fats, sugar, prescription drugs, and stress. To regain their stability, free radicals steal electrons from other molecules in your body, launching a domino effect that results in damage to your cells and your collagen. Free radicals are a certain path to visible signs of damage. The good news: antioxidants in Eat Pretty foods neutralize free radicals by giving them the electrons they seek and saving your beauty from harm.

An Avalanche of Oxidative Stress When there are too many free radicals in the body and not enough antioxidants to neutralize them, oxidative stress builds. Oxidative stress is the overall free-radical burden on your body. Growing levels of oxidative stress trigger inflammation, DNA damage, and mitochondrial slowdown—all major contributors to aging and damage that we'll explore in greater detail in the chapters ahead. There have also been studies exploring the connection between oxidative stress and graying hair, hair loss, and the aging of hair follicles—just one area where we see the un-pretty effects of stress!

Inflammation Fire Up Inflammation is a natural immune response triggered when the body sends white blood cells to the site of damage to begin healing. It's often characterized by heat, pain, and swelling, and it sparks blemishes, breakouts, redness, and wrinkles in the mirror. The far-reaching beauty effects of this un-pretty state have already earned a nickname—"inflamm-aging." Inflammation is also a contributing factor in dryness, itching, pain, even weight gain and depression. Sun exposure causes major inflammation in the skin, one reason that sunscreen is so important. But inflammation also occurs in our bodies as a response to our food choices, stress, lack of sleep, chemicals, even hormones. Inflammation is silent; it exists at a cellular level where you can't see or feel it, until it starts taking a toll on your beauty and health. Even low levels of inflammation show up as wrinkled, sagging skin if they're left unchecked, so lowering inflammation is one of the best strides you can take to preserve your beauty.

Unhealthy Acidity You've heard that pH balance is a plus when it comes to deodorant and shampoo, but did you know that a similar equilibrium between acidity and alkalinity is crucial in your very own internal chemistry? Most of your body needs a slightly alkaline pH for optimal beauty and health. Too many acidic foods (meat, dairy, sugar, caffeine) and habits (stress and lack of sleep) steal energy and nutrition from your body, speeding up the aging process, weakening bones, and causing dull, lackluster skin. You'll learn more on page 54.

Mitochondrial Burnout Feeling fatigued? Oxidative stress causes mitochondria, the powerhouses of our cells, to power down, which leaves our cells and organs lacking energy. We can protect our mitochondria by eating plenty of antioxidant-rich foods, as well as foods that are packed with the nutrients glutathione, manganese, vitamin C, CoQ10, alpha lipoic acid, and the amino acid L-carnitine. (The Beauty Nutrients chart on page 46, as well as the Eat Pretty food chapters in Part 2 of this book, will provide you with beautifying sources of these powerful compounds.) Another interesting tip: *too much* food stresses our mitochondria as well.

Overeating and lack of physical activity work together to stress our mito-chondria and contribute to metabolic syndrome, which causes high blood sugar and excess body fat storage around your middle and increases your risk for disease.

AGEs versus Age Healthy skin is supple, elastic, resilient, toned—but certainly not stiff. Advanced Glycation End Products, otherwise called AGEs, form in the body when excess sugars connect proteins, including structural proteins in your skin like collagen and elastin, creating stiff, rigid bonds. The result: wrinkling, sagging, and thinning. AGEs harm circulation by damaging blood vessels, contributing to a dull, dry com-plexion. They also create free radicals and inflammation in the body—as if you didn't have enough of those two to worry about! What's worse, AGEs don't just target your skin, they affect structural proteins in your muscles and bones, thus working to age you head to toe, inside and out-side. To support the health of your beauty and the longevity of your body, avoid the major causes of AGEs: high-glycemic foods that spike blood sugar, burned or overcooked foods, unprotected sun exposure, chemical additives in processed foods, smoking, and stress.

Confusing the DNA Blueprints DNA tells your cells how to act, how to build new parts, and what to do with the beauty nutri-tion you consume. But a diet lacking in good nutrition can in itself be a DNA stressor. In the pages ahead, you'll learn more about the exciting fields of nutritional genomics and epigenetics and just how profoundly our food choices influence our DNA and the state of our beauty and well-being. Eat Pretty nutrition protects the health of our DNA, which in turn preserves the strength and resilience of our beauty. All you need to remember is that swapping Beauty Betrayers for fresh, seasonal beauty foods sends your DNA the message to turn on your head-to-toe radiance.

THE INSIDE-OUT APPROACH

We're all guilty of choosing Beauty Betrayer foods that undermine our glow instead of Eat Pretty foods that support it. That's because much of the time we don't even realize we're making un-pretty choices! I spent years starving my skin, hair, and nails with a diet of processed foods that had the number of calories that I thought I needed, but no real beauty-supporting nutrition. When I didn't look or feel the way I wanted, I sought products that would cover my beauty issues from view. Such an outside-in approach to beauty pervades the daily images, practices, and habits of our culture—sometimes it feels like it's the only approach we know. But products are just a small part of the beauty equation. Judging by the millions of women who are frustrated with the beauty status quo, and the even greater numbers who just can't figure out how to look and feel their best, a superficial approach isn't working.

Take a look at the skin- and hair-care products on store shelves. You'll see an array of serums, lotions, and creams that protect skin from UV damage and deliver a layer of free radical–fighting antioxidants and other defensive compounds. But remember, these products are topical, so when they don't absorb well, get rubbed or rinsed away, wear off, or you just plain miss a spot, you're out of luck. In the worst-case scenario, products actually contribute to beauty issues with toxic ingredients that disrupt healthy hormone function and create inflammation. Antiaging products can be excellent age defense tools, but their effectiveness has limits; they block some outside attacks on our beauty, but leave us vulnerable to inside Beauty Betrayers. Many women don't know that they can boost their beauty by adjusting their diet, so they never try. But there is a simple formula for making a sweeping change: turning our approach inside out.

If this is your first encounter with the concept of beauty from the inside, I bet you're wondering why you didn't learn about the direct link between beauty and nutrition years ago. How is it that such a powerful shift in our understanding of beauty is happening only now? Beauty and nutrition are so clearly linked; yet in spite of powerful evidence, we've underestimated their relationship for decades. In some cases we under-valued, even misunderstood, the power of food, and in others we placed too much emphasis on outside beauty fixes. In the early part of the new millennium, fresh studies linking diet and acne emerged, and momen-tum built around the nutrition-beauty connection that applies to all of our beauty concerns, from acne and eczema to dull hair, weight gain, and wrinkles. Today we have scientific studies on record with data to show that sugar and dairy do contribute to breakouts; that fruits and vegetables make our skin look plumper and more hydrated; and that boosting our fruit and veggie intake actually makes us more attractive to others, by subtly altering the hue, and the glow, of our complexion.

Our understanding of inner beauty, like the saying "beauty is more than skin deep," has a long history, running across cultures and through centuries. But today our power to influence physical beauty from the inside is grounded in scientific fact, not only traditional wisdom. New findings in nutritional science, combined with our urgent need for a real solution to beauty issues like acne, weight gain, low energy, signs of aging, and loss of glow, make *this* the moment for change. But look around: during the decades-long dark ages in the realm of beauty nutrition, our routines were practically wiped clean of beauty-from-the-inside strategies. Eat Pretty helps you bring this wisdom back into focus by teaching you how to pamper and enhance your beauty at every meal and at every moment with the most up-to-date strategies.

If you feel ready to revitalize your beauty and body from the inside, let's change the way you think about every bite you take from this moment on. Consider this: the food you take in *becomes* your body, on a molecular level. This is one of the most momentous reasons that the quality of your diet is so critical to your beauty. Your breakfasts, lunches, snacks, and drinks contain the components of your muscle, your lymph, your bodily fluids, your skin cells, your sebum, and your bones. Your lunch doesn't enter and exit in a twenty-four- or even a forty-eight-hour period—those beauty nutrients stick around and become the raw materials that protect and repair your beauty from the outside attacks you experience in an average day. Would you choose to build and defend your body with the purest, cleanest, most potent beauty materials in nature, or low-quality ingredients that contain synthetic chemicals, dyes, and flavors? Of course you want only the best for your beauty and health! Eat Pretty foods provide the most powerful fuel for your beauty. If that's not enough to make you think twice about what you put on your plate, there's more; read on.

NUTRITIONAL GENOMICS AND EPIGENETICS

Exciting new research shows that our diet influences the instructions that our genes give to our bodies. Studies in nutritional genomics (the science relating diet and genetics) and epigenetics (the study of outside influences on our gene expression) confirm that we can switch our genes on and off with our food and lifestyle choices. No doubt you've heard buzz about these findings, but maybe their implications for your beauty weren't so clear.

While some components of food become the building blocks of our body, others end up in our bloodstream, where they influence genetic functions like the skin's ability to repair itself, the production of new collagen, and the regulation of inflammation. Quite likely you thought your genes were written in stone; that's true of your fixed genetic traits like the color of your eyes, the shape of your face, and the dimple on your left cheek. But we also have genes that are involved in the function of our systems—they tell your body how to make the keratin in your hair and nails, for example, or give the blueprint for building new skin cells and collagen day after day.

Genes, little segments of your DNA, contain the specific instructions for producing all the proteins in your body. You can't change your genes, but you can change the way they work in your body. This means turning off harmful genes, as well as turning on protective ones. Your diet and lifestyle choices influence as much as 80 percent of your genetic expression. This cutting-edge information shapes the Eat Pretty approach to beauty food.

So which foods exert the most beneficial and exciting influence over our gene activity? You'll be introduced to more than eighty-five of them in the pages ahead. But I can't help sharing a few delicious examples with you now. If you're looking for an instant beauty defender, the powerful antioxidant astaxanthin, present in wild-caught salmon, trout, and shrimp, protects the two outer layers of our cells from damage and shuts off inflammatory signals that lead to collagen breakdown. Need therapy for damage that's already been done? Delicate as its thin stems may seem, watercress has been shown in scientific study to repair DNA damage and increase our defenses against future DNA attacks. And like the age-old apple a day, science confirms that we receive beauty protection from the sweetness of pomegranates: their ellagic acid helps prevent aging inflammation in the body and turns off a cellular signal that breaks down collagen and sets the stage for wrinkles to form.

What we learn from studies in nutritional genomics and epigenetics will help us eat for even more specific beauty and antiaging effects in the years to come. Meanwhile, you shouldn't simply aim to eat three meals of salmon, watercress, and pomegranates every day; your body thrives on a diversity of nutrients, and your best beauty bet is to build your meals from a colorful and seasonal range of beauty foods. In Part 2 of this book, you'll read about my favorite beauty foods for each season of the year, plus the beauty food essentials for every pantry. While you should absolutely tailor your diet to your personal tastes, I passionately recommend that you sample as much of the full bounty of beauty foods catalogued herein as you can, since diversity and variety in your diet is the best way to take in an array of beauty nutrients. As you discover, or rediscover, these foods, you'll taste your most powerful sources of beauty, energy, health, weight management, and total radiance. You'll learn that food can pamper your body in its neediest moments and become your greatest support, rather than a daily source of damage and stress. Remember, you have control over your health, much more perhaps than you've been told or have come to feel. As you read *Eat Pretty*, remember that beauty is in your genes today; but it's how those genes perform that counts tomorrow. This is your opportunity to rewrite your genetic story.

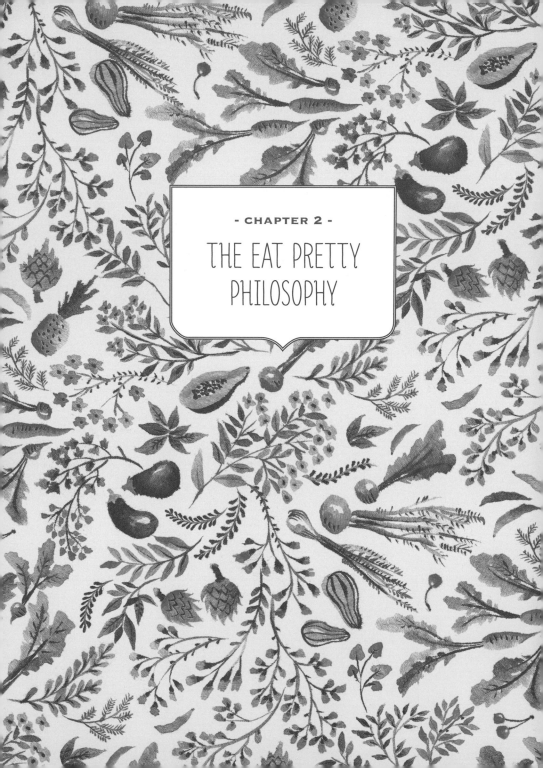

- CHAPTER 2 -

THE EAT PRETTY PHILOSOPHY

It's not simply a shortage of scientific research that kept us from adopting an inside-out approach to beauty in decades past; our learned relationships with food, our struggle to find beauty in ourselves, and the images of beauty that influence us daily all contribute to the lingering disconnect between beauty and nutrition. Eat Pretty helps you shift your thinking to see the big picture of beauty; you'll use this thinking to transform your life.

The essence of food, of course, is fuel. Every bite or sip you take delivers raw materials and, as you learned in the last chapter, powerful chemical messages that your body and beauty require to survive—and thrive. But food also has close ties to emotions, memories, celebrations, and comforts, and that complicates each and every food choice we make. Things get even more complex when outside influences make us feel that to be beautiful, we need to limit food or create strict patterns and rules around our eating habits. Take those influences to heart and you'll be misled into thinking that all food works against your beauty.

A BEAUTIFUL RELATIONSHIP WITH FOOD

There's no question: viewing food as only an enemy can age you beyond your years and seriously harm your beauty for decades to come. It's time to celebrate food as our most powerful beauty tool, not a detractor that makes us feel overweight or regretful. True, there are the Beauty Betrayer foods we met in Chapter 1; but you won't miss them, or the beauty issues like acne and wrinkles that they instigate. In the pages ahead, you'll learn to replace Beauty Betrayers with foods that enable you to look and feel your best. You'll realize that the foods we typically see as treats aren't treating us well in the least. So rethink how you splurge. Treat yourself to an expensive fillet of wild salmon or a basket brimming with organic produce. Your goal is to seek out the best foods for yourself. In them, you'll find beauty and health. Beauty foods are inherently those that make you feel good; they pack in the beautifying nutrients instead of packing on the pounds.

A word about getting off track: it happens to every single one of us. I didn't suddenly become a perfect eater when I found what I needed to change my body and beauty. I have days when I'm on a mission for a slice of greasy pizza, kale be damned. I love chocolate and wine and gluten-free cookies and cheese. But now I can feel when these foods are the wrong choices, and I know when my body is in danger of losing balance. Eat Pretty helped me listen to my body and appreciate what I need to look and feel my best. Learning to nourish my beauty from the inside gave me profound knowledge about myself that I will take with me during all stages of my life. This is the beauty wisdom that I want for you as well. Be kind to yourself as you learn it, and watch the beautiful transition in your life.

THE SOURCE OF BEAUTY

We measure our beauty in two major ways. The first, of course, is physical: the tone, clarity, and radiance of our skin; the strength of our nails; the thickness and shine of our hair; and even the scent that follows us into a room. Can you fake these things? A thousand times, yes. Plenty of us do so, every single day. This is the beauty that you can buy, and, sure, it'll get you by. There's a multi-billion-dollar industry built on helping us achieve greater physical beauty. Without it, I wouldn't have been able to hide my own skin troubles for years, and your favorite celebs wouldn't always look like living dolls on the red carpet. But it took me years to appreciate that, with only a one-sided view of good looks, I missed out not only on deeper physical beauty, but the other measure of beauty: the beauty we *feel*, as well.

Over the past several decades, we've adopted a fragmented approach to looking good. If your skin is dull, you need an exfoliant or a brightening lotion. If you have dark circles, apply an under-eye concealer. If your hair is thin and dry, use a conditioning mask. Our pieced-together beauty routines are in some ways very similar to conventional health-care diagnosis and treatment. Sometimes this highly specialized approach hits its target spot-on; other times it completely misses the big picture.

We need more "big picture" beauty. Thousands of products exist to treat our incredibly specific beauty concerns; at the same time, they distract us from looking more deeply at the root cause of these signs and symptoms. If we get too caught up in this world of product therapy, we may easily forget that our daily diet and lifestyle grant us major influence over the way our body and beauty behave—inside and out. Eat Pretty is a reminder that that your beauty isn't just a random set of independent parts. It's a total-body approach to good looks. Call it integrative beauty.

If you're like me, you've worked long and hard to find the products that fit you best, even if your routine is as spare as a swipe of lip balm and a dab of fragrance oil. These products work for you, and they make you feel great. I don't want you to give up any product that makes you feel beautiful (okay, unless it contains toxic ingredients—then swap it immediately). As long as the products in your routine make you feel fabulous and support your beauty with clean, safe ingredients, they are keepers! Without them, our beauty would be a lot less fun, a lot less colorful, and a lot less creative.

What Eat Pretty gives you that you can't get in a bottle or a tube is healthy groundwork. When you secure a beautiful foundation, you can take your look in whatever direction you choose. Beauty isn't in the color of the eyeshadow you wear today—it's in the radiant base underneath. When we strip away the layers of lipstick, powder, and primer and bring beauty back to its barest place, we see that the essential building blocks of beauty are the nutrients in the foods we take in each day. Our skin doesn't need antiaging serum to be healthy, but it absolutely cannot thrive without fats, protein, and essential nutrients like vitamins A, C, and E, zinc, and iron (you'll find details on these and other beauty nutrients in the next chapter). The same goes for our hair, nails, eyes, teeth, and bones. These nutrients are pure beauty fuel that gives our bodies the energy to defend, repair, renew, and fortify. Seizing their power is the key to a lifetime of gorgeous.

➢ FEELING BEAUTIFUL ⤾

Just as you can't limit your beauty routine to products and treatments alone, you can't talk about nurturing healthy vanity without including the central roles of lifestyle and emotional well-being. Nourishment takes many forms in your body. Beyond nutrition, beauty is fed with your breath, your thoughts, and the way you sleep, move, feel, and even digest. The big, big bonus of Eat Pretty is that it transforms another aspect of your beauty as well—your energy, vitality, mood, and emotions. This is the beauty that you feel. It isn't quite as tangible as your skin or hair, but I'd say it has an even stronger presence in your day-to-day life. You can totally fake this kind of beauty, too (how many times have you said, "I feel fine," when you really didn't?). But, unlike a lot of other things, if you continue to fake the way you feel, you'll never achieve the vibrant beauty that's within your reach. For a truly lasting beauty transformation, your body and mind must work together.

You're about to set out upon the path to total beauty, the kind that you can feel just as intensely as you see. Your food and drink offer energy and emotion to sustain you and build your beauty from the inside out. In a way, you ingest your feelings, so pause to identify your state of mind at mealtime and make it calm, focused, intentional, beautiful. Then take a moment to think about your appearance. What do you love most? What would you change? What signs have you noticed that tell you your beauty needs more support from within? You don't just shape your beauty when you're putting on or taking off makeup. Beauty is present in every breath and heartbeat—and bite. Your reward for embracing the Eat Pretty lifestyle is the ability to look better than you remember, even better than you can imagine, and create lasting change.

☙ FREE TO BE YOU ❧

The beauty nutrition guidelines in Eat Pretty are designed to make all of us glow from the inside out. But all of our bodies, while they march to some uniform laws of biology and chemistry, are different, too. We come from unique ethnic backgrounds, have different blood types, live in distinct environments, and generally have different likes and dislikes. So it's difficult to make any rule hard and fast. This book is veggie-rich; goes very light on dairy, gluten, and sugar; and recommends fish- and plant-based proteins. Use the information in these pages to create the beauty diet that supports you in the way that you need. Practice listening to your body's response to foods and habits—this will be one of your most valuable beauty skills. Everyone is a little different in their constitutions and their nutritional needs, and you'll learn to watch the way your body reacts to your choices. Raw foods, for example, are incredibly fresh and healthy, but all raw, all the time isn't suitable for many people. Learn to listen to your body's unique needs—and watch how those needs evolve.

If you're ready to transform your skin from the inside out, there's nothing holding you back; you can start your Eat Pretty lifestyle with your very next bite. With the right tools, you will look your best and feel better—tomorrow, as well as in the decades to come. You have the power to choose the foods that make you healthy, pretty, and vital. Don't be afraid to start small; small changes move mountains. They are the sustainable changes. Armed with your Eat Pretty knowledge, you won't feel like you're missing out when you swap a sugary latte and muffin for a breakfast of organic eggs and a green smoothie.

Start making Eat Pretty changes and you'll unequivocally feel more beautiful after just one meal. Balancing your blood sugar alone leads to a calm, steady mood and sustained energy, and, in the days to come, fewer breakouts and fine lines. Your skin, the first place to lose essential nutrients when they're needed elsewhere in the body, gets a fresh supply of nutrition after your first beautifying meal.

But don't stop at day one. In just three days of adopting Eat Pretty habits, you should see a brighter, more youthful complexion, since changes in your skin happen rapidly. Those changes will intensify in the weeks ahead, as your glow deepens and your skin develops better color, tone, clarity, and overall radiance. The whites of your eyes will be brighter and your body will feel lighter. It may take a bit longer to see the change in your hair and nails, but in about two months you will see a meaningful difference: strong, flexible nails free of ridges, splits, and white spots; pretty pink nail beds from well-oxygenated blood; glossy and strong hair that's less prone to thinning. This is the beauty that's universal, and it's accessible to all.

Remember, the journey you're beginning is more powerful than a quick fix. The changes you're making are new forms of pleasure and pampering, and building your beauty through nutrition and self-love is as thrilling as the good looks you set out to achieve. It's gorgeous that your beauty is a work in progress. Mine is too! I learn more about my body and beauty every day, and am constantly humbled by the wisdom and power of nature that fortifies and beautifies us daily. The seasons are a lesson to us. Our bodies are a lesson to us. The Eat Pretty approach to beauty is full of tools to help you boost your nutrition, restore balance to your life, and fulfill your beauty birthright. Your new mantra? "Beauty in, beauty out."

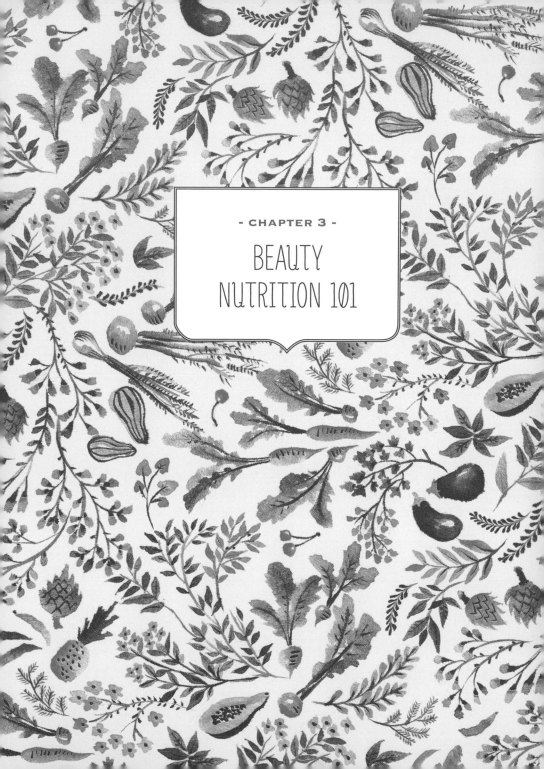

- CHAPTER 3 -

BEAUTY
NUTRITION 101

My job description hasn't changed much since my beauty editor days: I'm still here to give you the tools that make you look your best. Only I've had to rethink my toolkit. First on my must-have list: beauty nutrition. If you're ready to take a fresh look at food, you can launch your lifestyle of beauty from within at your next meal. When it comes to nutrition, Eat Pretty offers only the absolute best for you and your beauty. It's seasonal food that's colorful, whole, fresh, and allowed to ripen naturally for better taste and higher concentrations of beauty nutrients. It's quality over quantity. And it's exclusively the foods that support the way *you* want to look and feel. The foods on your plate are the most important beauty defenders you've got, so let's work up an appetite.

What is "pretty" food anyway? Far too many of us have the impression that any food that keeps us slim and beautiful is also tasteless and devoid of pleasure. But the foods and recipes that nourish your beauty from the inside aren't bitter pills to swallow—they're pleasure and pampering. I want you to savor them! The foods that keep you feeling great and fitting in skinny jeans aren't made with low-fat, sugar-free, or zero-calorie processed ingredients. Those ingredients *are* devoid of pleasure—for your taste buds and your beauty.

So many of the diets out there actually damage your beauty; they lack the protein your body needs to rebuild and repair, or they're deficient in good fats to keep your cells healthy and hydrated. They replace whole foods with processed bars and shakes that aim to quickly shed pounds—and starve your beauty in the process. At times they make you obsessive about what you can and cannot eat. Your body deserves a new approach, one that has the power to change you, cell by cell, from the inside out. That's how Eat Pretty works.

BUILDING BLOCKS OF BEAUTY

Let's warm up with the basics. You structure your meals from three major nutritional components: carbohydrates, fat, and protein. You should aim to eat the most beautifying examples of these types of foods every day, because not all carbs, fats, and proteins are created equal. Review the Beauty Betrayer foods (see pages 16 to 21) that sabotage healthy beauty until you know them by heart. It's possible to chow down on a burger and accurately argue that ground beef is your protein source, lettuce and a bun are your carbs, and mayonnaise and processed cheese are your fats. But in those types of carbs, fats, and protein, you also get hormones, pesticides, preservatives, and trans fats. They're inferior beauty fuel, instead of clean, high-quality building blocks for your beauty. The next section will guide you through the essentials in every Eat Pretty meal.

Carbohydrates Notorious "carbs" have been vilified by some diet plans, but there's no need to shy away from carbohydrates in general—just the Beauty Betrayers! The carbs to leave off your plate include processed cereals, chips, gluten-containing breads, soda, and refined desserts; these are the simple carbs that spike your blood sugar and burn up quickly, leaving you hungry for more. Complex carbs from vegetables, grains like oats and millet, and legumes like lentils digest slowly and cause less of a (blemish-triggering) spike in blood sugar. So go ahead and enjoy them, along with complex carb–packed sweet potatoes, beets, artichokes, peas, carrots, corn, and winter squash. Carbs are great energy sources for your body, and they provide ample vitamins, minerals, and fiber, as long as you choose Eat Pretty versions.

Fats Oh, how beauty suffered during the low-fat diet craze! Dull, lackluster skin, brittle hair and nails, cravings, and weight *gain* are some of the effects of a diet low in healthy fats. Today we know that healthy fats are essential for strong cell membranes; supple, well-hydrated skin;

and energy and nutrient absorption. Top-notch Eat Pretty fats are plant-based, unsaturated fats like olive and grapeseed oils, as well as coconut oil (a healthy saturated fat) and wild-caught fish and algae (sources of omega-3 fatty acids, the building blocks of fats). We need omega fatty acids in our diet because our bodies don't make them. Note that omega-6 fatty acids are already abundant in food, so focus on finding sources of omega-3s to include in your meals. They're found in salmon and sardines, as well as walnuts, chia seeds, shelled hemp seeds, and ground flaxseed.

Proteins If you want to grow strong collagen, elastin, and keratin—the components of youthful skin, hair, and nails—it's good to know who your friends are: lean, high-quality protein sources. Your skin alone is 25 percent protein. But don't think you need to be a meat eater to get gorgeous from the inside out. Eat Pretty encourages you to eat a variety of plant-based proteins, with the addition of some specific animal proteins like pastured eggs, wild salmon, sardines, and oysters. Varying the proteins in your diet is the best way to supply your body with a well-rounded supply of amino acids, the components that make up protein.

	FAVORITE EAT PRETTY SOURCES	BEAUTY BETRAYER SOURCES
Carbohydrates	Seasonal, organic vegetables and fruits; gluten-free grains; legumes	Refined sugar; soda; alcohol; processed cereals and snacks; gluten-containing grains, breads, and pastas
Fats	Coconut oil, olive oil, grapeseed oil, raw nuts and seeds, ground flaxseed, cold-water fish, avocados	Trans fats, fried foods, conventional dairy
Proteins	Algae and sea vegetables, sprouts, avocados, legumes, quinoa, raw nuts and seeds, pea and hemp protein, pastured eggs, wild salmon, sardines, oysters, tempeh	Conventional meat and dairy, egg substitutes, roasted nuts

Beauty Nutrition
GLOSSARY

Here are some common terms that will come up as we examine the amazing beauty benefits of Eat Pretty foods:

➢ **AMINO ACIDS** are the building blocks of proteins. They are some of the most important raw materials for your beauty, since they're essential for manufacturing and repairing healthy hair, nails, skin cells, and collagen, and they carry out instructions from your DNA to produce healthy beauty essentials like hormones and enzymes. The most critical amino acids in your diet are the nine essential amino acids that you must obtain from food. When you hear that a food is a "complete protein," you know it has all nine essential amino acids. Three of the key amino acids I mention in *Eat Pretty* are arginine, which boosts blood flow throughout the body (spinach, spirulina, and watermelon provide an arginine boost); glutamine, which heals and soothes the lining of the gut (beets, beans, spinach, and parsley are good sources); and tryptophan (found in beauty foods including pumpkin seeds, chickpeas, spirulina, bananas, and millet), which helps the body produce calming serotonin.

➢ **ANTIOXIDANTS** These powerhouse beauty nutrients give a missing electron to free-radical oxygen molecules that threaten to damage your beauty. (See page 22 for more on free radicals.) Antioxidants are the overarching name for many beautifying compounds in your foods, including nearly all phytochemicals, and some enzymes, vitamins, and minerals.

⚡ **ELECTROLYTES** are compounds that conduct electricity in our bodies to support the healthy function of our cells and organs. Some electrolytes come from minerals like potassium, sodium, and calcium.

⚡ **ENZYMES** are components of raw, living foods that speed up reactions and help your body function efficiently. They're especially beneficial to help your body digest foods and absorb beauty nutrients.

⚡ **FIBER** is the bulk prevalent in plant-based foods that keeps you full and satisfied. But it's more than just a placeholder in your digestive tract. Fiber detoxes the body, lowers cholesterol, promotes regular elimination, feeds healthy gut bacteria, and balances blood sugar.

⚡ **MINERALS** are inorganic chemical elements like magnesium, iron, and sodium that are essential for the healthy function of our beauty and body.

⚡ **PHYTOCHEMICALS** are chemical compounds found primarily in plant-based foods that deliver major beauty and health benefits.

⚡ **VITAMINS,** including the famous A, C, and E, are organic compounds in food that are essential for the healthy function of our beauty and body.

ASSEMBLING AN EAT PRETTY PLATE

To assemble a beautifying plate, you can include all three of the nutritional components discussed previously; or, using the food combining principles explained in Chapter 9, separate your proteins and your starchy carbs into different meals for optimal digestion. When you eat for beauty, the foundation of your meals should be seasonal, organic vegetables and fruits, especially the ones you'll read about in the chapters ahead. Add proteins and fats to your plate in smaller amounts. Always try to include vegetables and a small amount of healthy fats (which help you absorb beauty nutrients) at every meal. The exact quantity of carbs, fats, and protein you eat varies with your individual needs, and with different dietary theories and practices. But everyone should remember these key Eat Pretty concepts:

Wholeness. Beauty foods are whole foods, eaten in their most natural state. Choose foods that are of the highest quality, organic, and unrefined. Eat some raw when appropriate and cook others lightly—think living beauty fuel!

Color. Eating for beauty means choosing foods in a spectrum of vibrant hues. Natural color in vegetables and fruits signals high concentrations of antioxidant phytochemicals—plant chemicals that support healthy beauty. Remember to eat more of the natural reds, purples, greens, yellows, and blues, and less of the whites, beiges, and grays.

Variety. Eating the same foods every day, even if they're healthy and beautifying, leaves you in a nutritional rut. Broadening your food choices ensures that you get all of the different nutrients you need for healthy beauty. Let the seasons guide you. Eat seasonal vegetables and fruits and you'll enjoy the inherent wisdom of their nutritional benefits during every month of the year.

Anti-inflammation. We want our diet to *reduce* inflammation—which causes redness, dull skin, acne, and wrinkles and contributes to weight gain—not promote it, as the Beauty Betrayers do! The good news is that plant-based whole foods and healthy, uncooked fats are naturally anti-inflammatory.

Individuality. No single diet is right for everyone. Listen to your body, and take into account your environment and your specific dietary needs—like whether you have allergies, digestive difficulties, or deficiencies—while building your beautifying meals.

If there's a universal message here, it's that our food choices give us the power to reshape our beauty and body. Your body constantly remakes itself, even if it's not immediately apparent to your eyes, by producing new cells to replace those you lose. At this very moment your body is hard at work manufacturing millions of new cells. Antioxidants are neutralizing free radicals. Energy is being produced, and waste is being filtered. This is where your dietary choices become vital: nutrition is the tool that makes it all possible. You influence the quality of every cell in your body by choosing Eat Pretty foods that provide the nutritional blocks to build them stronger and more resilient. And at the same time you support the rebuilding and renewing of your assets, you create the defense system that will protect them for years to come. As you go about your day, your food choices fuel hundreds of important beauty functions. With inferior tools, these essential tasks won't be performed optimally—or at all—and your beauty will be the first place to suffer.

INSIDE YOUR BEAUTY FOODS

Pop quiz: name the important nutrients for beauty. Of course that's a trick question, since every single nutrient that supports the health of your body also supports a look-good, feel-good you. They *all* play a role, from the essential fatty acids to trace minerals like copper and phosphorus. And when you choose Eat Pretty sources of protein, fat, and carbs, you are filling your body with an abundance of beauty-boosting compounds that have a special ability to support your beauty from the inside. The nutrients outlined in the pages ahead have the power to supercharge your beauty and health, and they're all waiting for you in your Eat Pretty diet. Use the chart on the next page as your ultimate beauty nutrition reference.

BEAUTY NUTRIENTS
Your Healthy Beauty Must-Haves

NUTRIENT	BEAUTY BENEFITS	EAT PRETTY FOOD SOURCES
Vitamin A	• Essential for cell renewal and repair, and production of new skin cells, membranes, and tissues • Aids in cell turnover, to keep your skin smooth and glowing • Regulates the activity of the sebaceous (oil) glands • Important immune-booster • Extremely protective to our computer-strained eyes • Defends against UV damage to skin	Beet greens, butternut squash, carrots, collard greens, kale, pumpkin, romaine lettuce, spinach, sweet potatoes
Vitamin B$_1$/ thiamine	• Important for energy production • Supports nervous and digestive function	Black beans, Brussels sprouts, lentils, nuts, peas, sunflower seeds
Vitamin B$_2$/ riboflavin	• Aids in cell reproduction and growth	Mushrooms, pastured eggs, spinach, tempeh
Vitamin B$_3$/ niacin	• Keeps skin calm and moisturized • Essential for DNA repair	Asparagus, peas, sardines, wild salmon
Vitamin B$_5$/ pantothenic acid	• Helps maintain skin moisture • Keeps hair strong, with vibrant natural color	Avocado, mushrooms, pastured eggs, potatoes
Vitamin B$_6$/ pyridoxine	• Essential for regulating sleep, mood, and appetite • Prevents dry skin • Supports healthy hair color	Bananas, hazelnuts, pistachios, potatoes, spinach, sunflower seeds, wild salmon
Vitamin B$_7$/ biotin	• Powerful support for hair and nails • Nourishes adrenals • Essential for healthy metabolism	Almonds, avocado, chard, legumes, pastured eggs, wild salmon

NUTRIENT	BEAUTY BENEFITS	EAT PRETTY FOOD SOURCES
Vitamin B_9/ folate	• Helps repair cells and synthesize DNA • Essential for healthy pregnancy	Asparagus, Brussels sprouts, chickpeas, leafy greens, lentils, sprouts
Vitamin B_{12}*	• Important for metabolism, energy, and brain and nervous function	Oysters, pastured eggs, sardines, wild salmon
Vitamin C	• Essential for the production of collagen and elastin, structural components of skin that keep it toned and firm • Powerful antioxidant defender • Important for healthy metabolism • Regenerates vitamin E in the body	Bell peppers (red, orange, and yellow), Brussels sprouts, cabbage, kale, kiwi, papaya, pineapple, strawberries
Vitamin D**	• A mood booster that functions as a hormone once it builds up to a certain level in the body • Regulates the antimicrobial defenses of our skin • Essential for immunity, bone-building, and energy	Mushrooms, pastured eggs, sardines
Vitamin E	• Defends against free-radical damage • Maintains healthy, moisturized skin and scalp by protecting cell membranes and helping to build red blood cells • Supports healthy levels of antiaging glutathione	Almonds, avocados, chard, olives and olive oil, papaya, peaches, spinach, sunflower seeds, tomatoes
Vitamin K_1	• Important for healthy blood clotting • Strengthens blood vessels to reduce dark circles and prevent varicose veins	Asparagus, basil, beets, broccoli, Brussels sprouts, cauliflower, chard, collard greens, cucumber, escarole, kale, parsley, red cabbage, spinach

*   Vegetarians should talk to their doctor about supplementing vitamin B_{12}.
** Some other foods like almond milk are fortified with vitamin D, but it's generally hard to get enough from your diet. Talk to your doctor about supplementing with a high-quality vitamin D_3 capsule.

NUTRIENT	BEAUTY BENEFITS	EAT PRETTY FOOD SOURCES
Vitamin K_2	• Works with calcium to maintain healthy bones, teeth, and nails	Natto, some fermented vegetables
Alpha lipoic acid*	• Has hundreds of times more free radical-neutralizing potential than vitamins C and E combined • Protects our mitochondria and cells from aging • Aids in energy production • Reduces inflammation • Regenerates glutathione as well as vitamins C, E, and CoQ_{10} • May help reduce hormonal breakouts	Brewer's yeast, broccoli, spinach
Calcium	• Maintains strong and pretty teeth, bones, and nails • Regulates new skin cell production and wound repair • Calms nervous function	Acorn squash, almonds, Brazil nuts, broccoli, cabbage, chard, escarole, figs, kale, sardines, spinach
Copper	• Helps build bones and connective tissue • Supports healthy skin, hair, and nails • Produces melanin pigmentation in hair and skin • Important for nervous function	Apricots, cashews, chickpeas, coconut, goji berries, leafy greens, lentils, oysters, pineapple, potatoes, pumpkin seeds, tahini
CoQ_{10}	• Protects mitochondria from oxidative damage • Keeps cell membranes strong • Helps provide energy to cells • Defends against chronic fatigue and heart conditions • Supports healthy metabolism	Sesame seeds, walnuts

* For an additional source of alpha lipoic acid, talk to your doctor about supplementing.

Nutrient	Beauty Benefits	Eat Pretty Food Sources
Glutathione	• Powerful antioxidant • Protects your DNA by maintaining telomere length • Defends mitochondrial health • Boosts detox • Strengthens your immunity • Regenerates free radical–fighting vitamins C and E in the body	Artichokes, asparagus, avocado, beets, broccoli, cauliflower, cinnamon, collard greens, garlic, grapefruit, leeks, spinach, sprouts, turmeric, watercress, watermelon rind ← *EAT THE RIND*
Iodine	• Supports healthy thyroid function • Regulates metabolism	Sea vegetables like kelp, nori, wakame, and dulse
Iron	• Essential for the production of red blood cells, the transport of oxygen in the blood, and overall energy • Strengthens nails • Supports strong, shiny hair	Acorn squash, hemp seeds, kale, lentils, millet, oats, parsley, potatoes, pumpkin seeds, sea vegetables, spirulina, walnuts, watermelon
Magnesium	• Relaxes muscles • Reduces stress and PMS • Calms nervous function	Black beans, cashews, coconut, leafy greens, oatmeal, pumpkin seeds, quinoa, zucchini
Manganese	• Protects mitochondria • Helps maintain healthy hair and hair color • Aids in wound healing • Builds bones and connective tissue	Chickpeas, cinnamon, figs, green tea, oats, pecans, pineapple, potatoes, spinach
Omega fatty acids, including alpha-linolenic acid, linolenic acid, EPA, DHA	• Strong anti-inflammatory nutrients • Strengthen cell membranes and skin barrier • Aid in healthy oil production, for well-hydrated skin with fewer blackheads, and healthy scalp and hair • Assist in mood and hormone regulation • Important for brain and eye health	Algae, chia seeds, ground flaxseed, hemp seed, nori, sardines, trout, walnuts, wild salmon

NUTRIENT	BEAUTY BENEFITS	EAT PRETTY FOOD SOURCES
Phosphorus	• Maintains electrolyte balance • Aids in DNA repair and replication • Supports strong teeth, bones, and immune system	Broccoli, brown rice, burdock root, millet, potatoes, pumpkin seeds, quinoa, sardines
Potassium	• Important for healthy electrolyte balance and circulation • Supports healthy muscle and nerve function • Helps maintain pH balance in the body	Bananas, butternut squash, chard, potatoes, white beans
Probiotics	• Support healthy gut flora, which boost immunity, and help assimilate nutrients that nourish skin, hair, and nails • Aid in digestive function, which relieves gas and bloating • Encourage better elimination, taking a significant burden off of your skin	Fermented foods like miso, sauerkraut, and kimchi, or a probiotic supplement
Selenium	• Maintains skin elasticity • Protects against free-radical damage	Brazil nuts, coconut water, mushrooms, oats
Silicon	• Promotes strength and elasticity of skin and hair • Important for building collagen and strong connective tissues	Bananas, brown rice, burdock root, celery, cucumbers, leeks, oats, radishes, red cabbage
Sodium	• Maintains electrolyte balance • Supports nervous function	Miso, olives, oysters, sun-dried tomatoes
Sulfur	• Supports healthy hair	Arugula, cacao, garlic, radishes, red cabbage
Zinc	• Important for collagen formation and tissue healing • Helps regulate oil production • Fights inflammation and redness	Chia seeds, chickpeas, mushrooms, oysters, pecans, pumpkin seeds, quinoa, tahini, walnuts

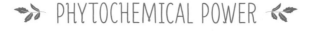

PHYTOCHEMICAL POWER

Phytochemicals are chemical compounds found primarily in plant-based foods that deliver major beauty and health benefits. They function differently from vitamins and minerals, but they're still some of your beauty's best friends. Each Eat Pretty food contains an assortment of unique phytochemicals that support your healthy beauty—there are thousands of phytochemicals in all. We won't get to discuss every one in this book, but we will cover the most valuable phytochemicals for beauty and antiaging. The chart below shows the benefits and sources of my favorite phytochemicals for beauty. Many of them, like curcumin, quercetin, and astaxanthin, are cutting-edge beauty boosters.

PHYTOCHEMICAL BEAUTY BOOSTERS
Nature's Bonus

PHYTOCHEMICAL		BEAUTY BENEFITS	EAT PRETTY FOOD SOURCES
Anthocyanins		• Boost skin elasticity • Protect DNA	Blueberries, cranberries, plums
Carotenoids	Astaxanthin	• Reduces DNA damage • Protects against sunburn	Wild salmon
	Beta-carotene	• Converts to vitamin A • Protects against UV damage	Apricots, beets, bell peppers, carrots, cherries, kale, papaya, sweet potatoes, tomatoes, winter squash
	Lutein	• Protects eye health	Chard, kale, pastured eggs, pumpkin, spinach

PHYTOCHEMICAL		BEAUTY BENEFITS	EAT PRETTY FOOD SOURCES
Carotenoids (continued)	Lycopene	• Defends against sun damage	Beets, grapefruit, papaya, tomatoes, watermelon
	Zeaxanthin	• Protects eye health	Apricots, kale, pastured eggs, pumpkin
Catechins	EGCG	• Fights free radicals	Green tea
	Epicatechin	• Blocks wrinkle formation	Cacao
Flavonoids	Gingerol	• Reduces inflammation • Defends against aging	Ginger
	Kaempferol	• Defends against cancer • Fights wrinkles	Endive, fennel, leeks
	Quercetin	• Blocks UVB damage • Reduces allergies	Apples, cherries, cranberries, fennel, green beans, onions, rhubarb
	Rutin	• Decreases AGE formation	Buckwheat
	Silymarin	• Supports liver and gallbladder health	Artichokes
Glucosinolates	Allicin	• Blocks wrinkle formation • May be cancer-preventative	Garlic, leeks, onions
	Indole-3-Carbinol	• Reduces the risk of estrogen-sensitive cancers • Helps balance hormones	Broccoli, Brussels sprouts, cabbage

PHYTOCHEMICAL		BEAUTY BENEFITS	EAT PRETTY FOOD SOURCES
Glucosinolates (continued)	Sulforaphane	• Reduces inflammation • Reduces redness from UV exposure • Boosts glutathione	Broccoli, broccoli sprouts, cauliflower, kohlrabi, turnips, watercress
Phenolic Acids	Capsaicin	• Blocks wrinkles • Reduces inflammation	Cayenne, chile peppers
	Curcumin	• Reduces inflammation • Reduces pain	Turmeric
	Ellagic Acid	• Blocks wrinkles • Aids in blood sugar balance	Pecans, pomegranates, raspberries, strawberries
Other	Betalain	• Boosts glutathione production	Beets
	Chlorophyll	• Oxygenates blood • Detoxifies metals • Feeds good bacteria in the gut	Cucumber, leafy greens, parsley
	Coumarin	• Lowers blood pressure	Celery
	Lignan	• Supports healthy digestion • May help prevent breast cancer	Ground flaxseed
	Resveratrol	• Activates sirtuin genes that turn on reparative, protective enzymes	Raspberries, red grapes with seeds

Beauty in BALANCE

You've just learned about essential beauty nutrients, but there's yet another way to assess the beautifying potential of your foods: in their acid or alkaline effect on your body. At any given moment there are dozens of chemical processes happening inside you, sans test tubes and beakers, and your body's pH (potential of hydrogen, a measure of acidity and alkalinity) influences the environment where they all take place. Most of your internal environment is healthiest at or near a slightly alkaline pH, and when too many acidic foods enter your body, your internal fluids threaten to stray beyond a very small alkaline pH window, and your body immediately takes action to maintain its pH level. The body goes so far as to steal energy and beautifying nutrients that should be put to use for other tasks (like making sure you look your best) in order to keep you balanced.

Acidity shows up in the mirror as exhaustion—exhausted skin, exhausted body, plus dry and lackluster hair and a dull, drawn complexion. With an acidic diet, you might also see an increase in blemishes and redness, since acidity and inflammation go hand in hand, speeding up aging and stealing from your natural glow and vitality. Acidic foods rob essential beauty minerals and aggravate existing acne and weight issues by adding to your body's overall beauty burden. Eating more alkaline foods, on the other hand, boosts your immunity and encourages weight loss by easing the waste removal process. So where can you get more of these alkaline superfoods? Most fruits (even citrus!), vegetables, and spices are alkaline because they contain high levels of minerals. Foods high in sugar, caffeine, and chemical additives are acid-forming in the body, as are most grains, nuts, meats, dairy, and oils. Fresh, seasonal, alkaline foods are the core of Eat Pretty—another reason to build your next meal from the beauty foods you'll find ahead.

PRETTY IN A PILL

If you stock up on multivitamins and a few other supplements, you could check off your daily beauty nutrient needs in a few big swallows, right? In a way, yes, *but* . . . the bottom line is, it's always best to get your nutrition from whole foods first. Quite often we hear of studies about antioxidants or other compounds isolated from foods, and we try to consume them in concentrated doses. Don't be thrown off track by that reductionist approach. Your foods provide unique compositions of vitamins, minerals, amino acids, phytochemicals, and other compounds that work synergistically; supplements can't always replicate their benefits. Rather than try to pinpoint specific nutritional deficiencies, I urge you to build your Eat Pretty diet around well-rounded health. Always start with whole foods, which in their natural state combine complementary nutrients, allowing you to digest, absorb, and utilize the nutrients that you're seeking. For example, we miss out on the beauty benefits of egg yolks, with their lutein and zeaxanthin antioxidants, healthy fatty acids, and plant-based progesterone, when we only eat the whites. In Eat Pretty, we favor the whole: the whole plant, the whole food, and the whole you.

NUTRITION IN THE KITCHEN

Let's move on to Part 2, where you'll build your Eat Pretty pantry and fill your kitchen with the freshest, most vibrant foods from each season. You'll learn to create a lifestyle of beauty and pampering at any time of the year with deeply nourishing foods and recipes. "Let food be thy medicine and medicine be thy food," said the Greek physician Hippocrates, to which I'd add, let food be your beauty secret as well. Read on to blend, juice, chop, and taste your way to radiant beauty, and the seasonal secrets that I can't wait to share.

PART 2

FOUR SEASONS
TO EAT PRETTY

The transformation in the way you look and feel actually starts with a makeover for your pantry, your fridge, and your kitchen cabinets. In the pages ahead, I'll take you through the most important ingredients to stock in your beauty kitchen, so you'll always be prepared to create an Eat Pretty meal. Then we'll move on to the four seasons, each with its own season-specific beauty intentions and a basketful of beauty foods to savor. The accompanying recipes and beauty editor tips will give you a peek at my favorite ways to live an Eat Pretty lifestyle throughout the year. As you nourish your body with these seasonal Eat Pretty foods, you'll see the potential to bring beauty into every choice you make. What is your next bite going to do for your hair? How about your mood? Or your skin? Does it support *you*? Your Eat Pretty knowledge is your power, and your healthy vanity is your motivation. Together they lead you to a more beautiful life—and the most beautiful you. Your beauty transformation starts with your next bite, so make it a delicious one!

CHAPTER 4

A BEAUTIFUL KITCHEN
FOR ALL SEASONS

If I asked you to run to your beauty cabinet and bring me your top two beauty tools, would you come back with a serum and an eye cream? Or a vitamin-infused cuticle oil and a deep conditioner? By now, I bet you think differently about beauty tools. In your Eat Pretty lifestyle, your beauty command center isn't in the bathroom or at your vanity—it's in your kitchen. Your cabinets should be stocked with advanced nutritional weaponry to keep you looking healthy and gorgeous from the inside out. Even if you're short on time to bake, chop, and sauté, getting smart about how you stock your kitchen will spark a major change in the way you look and feel.

➢ YOUR EAT PRETTY JUMPSTART ‹‹

Ready to assemble your edible beauty supplies? You'll need a quick make-over for your kitchen: first, to clear space for the seasonal beauty foods and pantry staples you're going to dive into in the following chapters; and, second, to make it as easy as possible for you to choose beautifying foods every day. If you have a refrigerator that's completely bare except for a few condiments and a bottle of wine, then there's already plenty of room for beauty foods—you're set! But if your cabinets are brimming with packaged snacks and sweets, processed meats, dairy products, and sugary sodas and juices that don't support your beauty, take this moment to make space on your shelves, and in your life. Clear out your favorite cabinet and start fresh. Scratch Beauty Betrayer foods off this week's grocery list and toss as many of them as you can. It sounds wasteful, but you're throwing away foods that actually damage your beauty and your health. You're so much more gorgeous without them!

One thing I don't want is for you to feel absolutely frozen with dread about throwing away your favorite foods. That fear causes stress, which, as you'll learn in Part 3, is as big a saboteur of beauty as any Beauty Betrayer food. I won't send you into a panic by forcing any one food from your life. It's normal, healthy, and beautiful to splurge now and then, if you are truly honoring your body and beauty. Be honest, though—if you keep Beauty Betrayer foods like chips, cookies, candy, and soda within reach, the splurge won't be *occasional*. Even if you work hard to be a beautiful eater, the presence of those un-pretty foods can tempt you when you least expect it. If you choose to save room in your cabinets for Beauty Betrayers, know that you'll be able to see and feel their effects every time you eat them. I challenge you to start with a clean slate to achieve the most stunning results from your Eat Pretty diet.

The Eat Pretty
⤳ PANTRY ↢

Not making time to cook for myself was one of my biggest beauty blunders. Learning to cook daily meals helped me truly care about my diet, and it became the core of my Eat Pretty transformation. Even though I always loved to cook, preparing a meal for one felt like a wasted effort, and I was exhausted every day after work anyway. I also never had the beauty food pantry staples I needed to build a beautifying meal—and that's half the battle. Don't you fall prey to an empty-pantry takeout binge, too! I'm about to help you stock a powerful beauty kitchen. Every item in the list ahead is brimming with beauty benefits, and it'll keep well on your shelves until you find the perfect moment to pull it out to cook yourself a meal that helps you look and feel your best. For more information on the beauty nutrients in the following foods, refer to the Beauty Nutrients chart (page 46) and Phytochemical Beauty Boosters chart (page 51).

ALMOND MILK: Healthy Skin Drink

Coconut and hemp non-dairy milks also nourish your beauty, but in my book unsweetened almond milk wins for flavor and skin benefits. Plain almond milk found in your supermarket is usually fortified, so when you pour a cup or so over your oatmeal, you get about half of your daily dose of vitamin E, the beauty vitamin that keeps skin moisturized and protected from the sun, plus about 45 percent of your calcium and 25 percent of your vitamin D. Unsweetened almond milk is low in both sugar and calories, and it's free of the hormones and antibiotics found in conventional dairy.

EAT PRETTY FOOD	BEAUTIFYING COMPOUND	BEAUTY BENEFIT
Almond milk (unsweetened)	Vitamin E	Boosts skin moisture

APPLE CIDER VINEGAR: pH Balancer

Apple cider vinegar may taste acidic on your tongue, but it's highly alkaline, so it balances acidic foods in your body to maintain a healthy pH (see page 54). Apple cider vinegar is a wonderful digestive tonic that prevents constipation (easing the waste-eliminating burden on your skin) and wards off bad bacteria. It also increases the acidity of the stomach, important since many of us have digestive troubles from low stomach acid. Apple cider vinegar also contains potassium and a detoxifying fiber called pectin. Vinegar of all types steadies your blood sugar by slowing the digestion of carbs, thanks to acetic acid. Buy the raw, unrefined version of apple cider vinegar (I love it in homemade dressings) to get the most potent beauty benefits.

EAT PRETTY FOOD	BEAUTIFYING COMPOUND	BEAUTY BENEFIT
Apple cider vinegar	Potassium	Maintains pH balance

BEE POLLEN: Buzz-Worthy Beauty Food

These tiny pollen granules are packed with nutrients that support your beauty and your energy. Bee pollen is a complete protein source, with twenty-two amino acids that are essential for the production of new skin cells, not to mention keratin, for gorgeous hair and nails. Bee pollen is also a concentrated source of energy-boosting B complex vitamins. Bee pollen is used as a remedy for allergies, since it contains the anti-histaminic phytochemical quercetin, as well as for digestive issues, since it's rich in enzymes that ease the digestive burden on our bodies. Sprinkle a small amount of bee pollen into smoothies and onto salads and desserts.

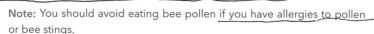

> Note: You should avoid eating bee pollen if you have allergies to pollen or bee stings.

EAT PRETTY FOOD	BEAUTIFYING COMPOUND	BEAUTY BENEFIT
Bee pollen	Enzymes	Support healthy digestion

BUCKWHEAT: Youthful Skin Protector

Nutty, savory buckwheat is not wheat at all—it's a member of the rhubarb family. I love cooking with both buckwheat flour and the whole grains, called groats. Buckwheat's main phytochemical, rutin, decreases the formation of wrinkle-promoting AGEs in the body, making it a major antiaging beauty food. Buckwheat flour is gluten-free and a nutritious alternative to white flour, thanks to its lower glycemic index and high levels of iron, magnesium, protein (including essential amino acids), and fiber. Store your buckwheat flour in the fridge or freezer to keep its high content of healthy oils at peak freshness.

EAT PRETTY FOOD	BEAUTIFYING COMPOUND	BEAUTY BENEFIT
Buckwheat	Rutin	Decreases wrinkle-forming AGEs

CHIA SEEDS: Omega Powerhouse

If you haven't caught on to the powerful benefits of chia seeds, it's time to add this tiny superfood to your beauty cabinet. Chia seeds are a great source of cell-strengthening omega-3 fatty acids that reduce inflammation and protect the skin from sun damage. Chia seeds are a complete protein (those amino acids are crucial for healthy skin, hair, and nails) and they're a good source of bone-building calcium and zinc, for blemish-free skin. Chia seeds are packed with soluble fiber that improves elimination and reduces bloating while making you feel fuller with fewer calories. Create your own chia-seed pudding by combining a scoop of chia seeds and enough almond milk to cover until the seeds form a gelatinous outer layer—it's an easy detox recipe!

EAT PRETTY FOOD	BEAUTIFYING COMPOUND	BEAUTY BENEFIT
Chia seeds	Omega-3s	Strengthen skin cells

CHICKPEAS: Clear Skin Secrets

Chickpeas (also called garbanzo beans) are antioxidant-rich legumes full of phytochemicals that boost immunity and aid in the absorption of other important beauty minerals. They pack in the protein, fiber, folate, and trace minerals like zinc, the antioxidant beauty mineral that keeps skin clear and scalp healthy and promotes hair growth and strong nails. Chickpeas also contain copper and manganese, two important minerals for healthy, energetic, and youthful cells. Chickpeas are a fiber-rich source of complex carbohydrates that stabilize your blood sugar levels, staving off wrinkles and hormonal imbalance.

EAT PRETTY FOOD	BEAUTIFYING COMPOUND	BEAUTY BENEFIT
Chickpeas	Zinc	Supports clear skin

✓ COCONUT OIL: Metabolism Booster

Coconut oil will change what you think about fats. It's made of anti-inflammatory, medium-chain fatty acids that burn quickly and easily in the body without being broken down by the liver, providing instant energy and a metabolism boost that actually helps us burn stored fat. Of course that doesn't give you a pass to overindulge. Use a teaspoon or two in a stir-fry (it's stable at high heat and won't produce free radicals) or baked goods, and add a little to smoothies, since coconut oil actually boosts your absorption of other nutrients.

The main component of coconut oil is lauric acid, a powerful anti-microbial fat that kills bacteria, viruses, and yeast (it's also found in breast milk!). Coconut oil is saturated, so it's solid at room temperature, but won't harm your cholesterol—it actually lowers LDL (bad cholesterol) and raises HDL (good cholesterol) in the body. Saturated fats like coconut oil are essential for healthy cell membranes and gorgeous skin.

EAT PRETTY FOOD	BEAUTIFYING COMPOUND	BEAUTY BENEFIT
Coconut oil	Lauric acid	Supports metabolism and fat burning

✓ FLAXSEED: Omega Wonder

Flaxseed is full of phytochemicals called lignans that aid digestion and may help prevent breast cancer, thanks to their ability to mimic estrogens in the body. Ground flaxseed is an excellent plant source of anti-inflammatory omega-3s, especially alpha-linolenic acid, an essential fatty acid that the body converts to eicosapentaenoic acid (EPA)—the same fat-burning, collagen-boosting omega-3 found in fish oil. Omega-3s decrease levels of a hormone that can be a factor in clogged pores and breakouts, and they ensure that your skin is healthy enough to retain moisture. Add ground flaxseed to your meals for extra fiber that supports healthy elimination, and protein for skin-damage repair.

EAT PRETTY FOOD	BEAUTIFYING COMPOUND	BEAUTY BENEFIT
Flaxseed	Alpha-linolenic acid	Reduces inflammation

GOJI BERRIES: The Youth Fruit

These little red berries are sometimes called the "longevity fruit," and with good reason: The amino acid glutamine in goji berries stimulates the body's production of HGH, a hormone partially responsible for the youthful appearance and fast healing ability that declines with age. Glutamine in gojis also aids in the production of glutathione, the body's master antiaging nutrient. Goji berries have the exceptional ability to defend mitochondrial health and protect against DNA damage. They also contain eighteen amino acids, as well as beauty minerals like iron, zinc, and copper, for gorgeous skin, hair, and nails. Try them in trail mix or hot cereal.

EAT PRETTY FOOD	BEAUTIFYING COMPOUND	BEAUTY BENEFIT
Goji berries	Glutamine	Supports antiaging HGH and glutathione production

HEMP SEEDS: Omega Beauty Love

Shelled hemp seeds are a complete source of protein that support cell building and repair, for enviable skin, hair, and nails. They are an excellent source of anti-inflammatory, antiaging omega fatty acids, including gamma-linolenic acid, an important fat for healthy skin and the healing of eczema. Hemp seeds have lots of fiber for healthy elimination, as well as iron and zinc—more good news for your beauty. I love adding them to smoothies, hot cereals, salads, and desserts for a soft, nutty crunch.

EAT PRETTY FOOD	BEAUTIFYING COMPOUND	BEAUTY BENEFIT
Hemp seeds	Gamma-linolenic acid	Helps heal eczema

LENTILS: Protein Powerhouses

Lentils are my favorite beautifying legumes, for their excellent protein content and blood sugar-stabilizing energy. Both protein and blood sugar stability are key for healthy, wrinkle-free, clear skin. Lentils are incredibly rich in folate, an important nutrient for DNA synthesis and cell repair, as well as iron for strong nails. Bonus: they're relatively quick cooking and don't need soaking! Store lentils, along with your other beautifying grains and beans, at eye level in pretty jars so you'll always be inspired to use them.

EAT PRETTY FOOD	BEAUTIFYING COMPOUND	BEAUTY BENEFIT
Lentils	Folate	Supports cellular repair

MILLET: Seed of Happiness

This light, fluffy, gluten-free seed (we cook it like a grain) is rich in amino acids that support cell maintenance and repair. Millet is an alkaline seed that's a rich source of beauty minerals, including iron for healthy hair and nails, magnesium for gorgeous teeth and bones, manganese to protect the mitochondria, and phosphorus for DNA repair. The amino acid tryptophan in millet gets converted to feel-good serotonin in the body, <u>keeping you happy and calm</u>. Millet is also full of fiber that fills you up, maintains blood sugar stability, and feeds healthy bacteria in your digestive system.

EAT PRETTY FOOD	BEAUTIFYING COMPOUND	BEAUTY BENEFIT
Millet	Tryptophan	Supports mood-boosting serotonin

✓ NUTS: Beauty Builders

Nuts are little nuggets of healthy fats, protein, and beauty minerals that fill you up, sustain you, and travel easily, making them ideal beauty foods for our busy lives. The selection of nuts in your pantry might change with your mood or with the seasons, so let your taste buds guide you. Almonds are rich in vitamin E, for strong cell membranes and wrinkle prevention. Cashews are full of copper, which contributes to radiant hair pigmentation. Pistachios pack in the B$_6$ for healthy, oxygenated blood. Brazil nuts are major sources of selenium, which helps maintain skin elasticity and the body's production of glutathione.

Always buy your nuts organic and raw, since roasted nuts often contain oxidized oils that create age-advancing free radicals and AGEs, while the heathy fats in raw nuts reduce inflammation in the body. Before you snack on raw nuts, it's best to soak them for a couple of hours or up to overnight to release their enzyme inhibitors and make them more easily digestible. Store them in a cool, dark place or in the refrigerator or freezer if you won't use them quickly.

EAT PRETTY FOOD	BEAUTIFYING COMPOUND	BEAUTY BENEFIT
Raw nuts	Healthy fats	Reduce inflammation

OATS: Morning Dose of Beauty Minerals

Oats are <u>mineral-rich breakfast staples</u>. They're extremely high in manganese, which helps maintain healthy hair and hair color and supports mitochondrial health. They're also rich in the beauty mineral iron, for strong hair and nails. Oats are high in antiaging selenium—a powerful nutrient for skin elasticity and production of champion antioxidant glutathione—and vitamin B₁, instrumental in healthy nervous system function. For the most beauty benefits, buy gluten-free oats. If not specifically labeled "gluten-free," oats usually pick up gluten during processing in the same facilities as wheat.

EAT PRETTY FOOD	BEAUTIFYING COMPOUND	BEAUTY BENEFIT
Oats	Manganese	Supports healthy hair and hair color

OLIVE OIL: Sensitive Skin Secret

Stock your kitchen with extra-virgin olive oil for a major dose of antioxidants that keep your skin looking supple and youthful. A moderate amount of olive oil in your diet can help maintain a trimmer waistline, reduce the risk of heart disease and high blood pressure, and raise good HDL cholesterol levels. Olive oil is anti-inflammatory (great for calming sensitive skin) and rich in vitamin E, a UV-protective vitamin that strengthens cell membranes and works in tandem with vitamin C to provide a fantastic defense against aging. For the biggest beauty benefits, it's best to save olive oil for topping salads, dips, and vegetables after they're cooked; use coconut oil for your high-heat cooking to avoid forming free radicals.

EAT PRETTY FOOD	BEAUTIFYING COMPOUND	BEAUTY BENEFIT
Olive oil	Vitamin E	Defends against UV damage

POPCORN: Antioxidant-Rich Snack

Organic popcorn hulls are packed with free radical–fighting phytochemicals, but before you dive into a bowl, there's one caveat: you need to toss out your microwave popcorn bags (they're loaded with artificial flavors and chemicals) and stick to plain popcorn kernels, which you can pop easily on the stovetop or in a brown paper bag in the microwave. Air-popped popcorn is a beautifying snack because it fills you up with minimal calories (about 15 in one handful) and lots of fiber. To make air-popped popcorn even more of an Eat Pretty food, add a topping like nutritional yeast, melted dark chocolate, or antioxidant spices such as cinnamon, turmeric, or cayenne.

EAT PRETTY FOOD	BEAUTIFYING COMPOUND	BEAUTY BENEFIT
Popcorn	Fiber	Promotes healthy elimination

The Forgotten BEAUTY NUTRIENT

There is one health essential that isn't actually a nutrient, but still has tons of beauty power: water. Water makes up 60 to 70 percent of our body weight and 70 percent of our skin, but it's usually pretty low on our list of health priorities. Having interviewed my share of models through the years, I'd say that "Drink water" is their quintessential skin secret. Plenty of people shrug off hydration as obvious, but there's some real science to pay attention to here. Dehydration releases stress hormones, which in turn leads to an increase in aging inflammation in the body. Water is also essential for bodily functions from metabolism and nutrient absorption (key for water-soluble nutrients like vitamin B complex and vitamin C) to detoxification, circulation, and temperature regulation. The body hydrates more efficiently when we eat (rather than drink) some of our water, too, as in water-rich foods like watermelon, cucumber, apple, and celery that slowly hydrate as they make their way through our digestive system.

QUINOA: Complete Beauty Protein

A complete protein that's not animal based? Meet quinoa, your new beauty BFF. Quinoa has all nine essential amino acids, which build strong, youthful skin, hair, and nails and repair daily damage. Quinoa is actually a seed, one that's gluten-free and nutrition-packed like its relative, spinach. In addition to its powerful protein content, quinoa is full of trace beauty minerals like iron, zinc, magnesium, manganese, and phosphorus. Its complex carbohydrates and low glycemic index steady your blood sugar and keep you full, yet free of bloating. Quinoa also supports healthy digestion with fiber that feeds healthy bacteria in your intestines.

EAT PRETTY FOOD	BEAUTIFYING COMPOUND	BEAUTY BENEFIT
Quinoa	Protein	Aids in cell growth and repair

SARDINES: Small Fish, Big Beauty

Sardines, while small, are one of the biggest fish in the sea when it comes to beauty. They're full of anti-inflammatory, beauty-boosting omega-3s like EPA, one of the omega-3 fats in fish that has been shown to preserve collagen and amp up fat burning. Omega-3s decrease the levels of a hormone that has been linked to excess sebum and clogged pores—two big blemish-causers. Sardines are high in selenium, an essential mineral that keeps skin firm and repairs damage. They contain vitamin D to maintain strong bones and prevent sagging and wrinkling skin caused by bone loss. In the fish world, where levels of metals and other toxins can be a concern, sardines rank high on the list of the cleanest fish to eat. Try protein-packed sardines in the morning to keep your energy and blood sugar steady for hours.

EAT PRETTY FOOD	BEAUTIFYING COMPOUND	BEAUTY BENEFIT
Sardines	Omega-3s	Reduce inflammation

spirulina - pond scum!
wakame - seaweed
kelp seaweed
dulse - alga _kombu - seaweed_
edible algae/seaweed

SEA VEGETABLES: _Beauty Mineral Magic_

Sea vegetables are simply incredible for beauty. Take nori, the humble sushi sheet: it's packed with omega-3s (more than olive oil or a whole avocado) and trace minerals that feed your skin, hair, and nails, plus it's more than 50 percent pure protein. But nori's just the starter sea veggie. Sea plants like wakame, spirulina, kelp, dulse, and kombu also deserve a place in your Eat Pretty pantry. Try kelp flakes on your salads and veggies, or spirulina powder for extra protein and minerals in smoothies. The beauty mineral benefits of sea veggies are potent, even in very small doses.

Note: Iodine in sea vegetables can help support healthy thyroid function, but talk to your doctor about eating iodine-rich foods if you already have a thyroid condition.

EAT PRETTY FOOD	BEAUTIFYING COMPOUND	BEAUTY BENEFIT
Sea vegetables	Iodine	Regulates metabolism

✓ EAT PRETTY SWEETENERS: _Sweet and Skin-Friendly_

Stock your Eat Pretty pantry with healthier sweeteners to reduce your intake of refined sugar, a big Beauty Betrayer. My favorite sweeteners are stevia, maple syrup, raw honey, coconut sugar, and blackstrap molasses, which have beauty benefits and a lower glycemic index than refined sugar (but should still be eaten in moderation!). Stevia is several hundred times sweeter than sugar, has no calories, and may actually improve insulin sensitivity. It does leave a bit of an aftertaste, so I combine it with other sweeteners to amplify their sweetness. Maple syrup contains trace minerals like zinc, iron, and manganese, plus it's anti-inflammatory. Raw honey is filled with active enzymes, B vitamins, minerals, and antibacterial properties—but it must stay unheated to retain these properties (so don't add it to boiling hot tea). Coconut sugar is minimally processed and low glycemic, and it contains B vitamins and potassium. Blackstrap molasses is rich in iron, and it

Glow-Getters:
ANTIAGING HERBS AND SPICES

Parsley, sage, rosemary, and thyme— and ginger and cumin and cloves: You can't go wrong with the beauty benefits of fresh herbs and spices. Spicing up your meals could be the easiest way to amplify their beautifying benefits. Here are sixteen of the essential herbs and spices in my Eat Pretty pantry:

- ✓ **BASIL** contains flavonoids that protect your cells from oxidative damage.
- **CARDAMOM** relieves indigestion and detoxifies the body.
- **CAYENNE** boosts immunity and metabolism, and helps curb cravings.
- ✓ **CINNAMON** keeps blood sugar steady, preventing insulin spikes that lead to wrinkles and blemishes.
- **CLOVES** aid in digestion and contain a strong anti-inflammatory oil.
- **CUMIN** is a good source of iron and a digestive booster.
- **FENNEL SEEDS** are high in the UVB-protective phytochemical quercetin.
- ✓ **GINGER** is a proven reliever of muscular aches and pains brought on by exercise.
- **MINT** eases indigestion and promotes detox.
- ✓ **NUTMEG** helps you achieve more restful beauty sleep.
- ✓ **OREGANO** has antioxidant, antimicrobial properties that make it a popular cold-fighter.
- ✓ **PARSLEY** is packed with iron and is a blood cleanser.
- **ROSEMARY** boosts mood and memory.
- **SAGE** helps regulate bile flow for healthy digestion.
- **THYME** contains powerful antioxidant, anti-inflammatory compounds.
- **TURMERIC** reduces inflammatory pain and speeds up healing.

imparts great flavor to holiday sweets and savory dishes. Try one, or all, in your kitchen as a replacement for table sugar.

EAT PRETTY FOOD	BEAUTIFYING COMPOUND	BEAUTY BENEFIT
Stevia, maple syrup, raw honey, coconut sugar, blackstrap molasses	Unrefined sugar	Prevents the high insulin spike of refined white sugar

TAHINI: Skin and Hair Booster - major ingredient in Hummus

Tahini, a thick, oily paste of ground sesame seeds, is a Middle Eastern staple and a beautifying food that adds an earthy flavor to dressings, dips, and smoothies. It's rich in essential beauty minerals like zinc and calcium that keep skin, scalp, hair, and nails healthy, and it contains essential omega-3 fats that nourish healthy cell membranes. Another major beauty benefit of tahini: its stress-busting B vitamins keep our nerves at ease. The less we stress, the more we lessen the aging burden on our body.

EAT PRETTY FOOD	BEAUTIFYING COMPOUND	BEAUTY BENEFIT
Tahini	Zinc	Supports clear skin

JUST ADD VEGGIES

With these versatile ingredients stocked in your beauty kitchen, you'll never need to hit up the drive-thru for an order of Beauty Betrayers on your way home. Instead, bring home seasonal fruits and vegetables and combine them with your Eat Pretty pantry foods for a no-fuss meal that supports radiant skin, silky hair, strong nails, a healthy weight, and good moods. If you need beautifying recipe ideas, you'll find twenty in the pages ahead. And while the beauty foods in your pantry might be the same all year, the fresh foods you'll find at the market change with the seasons. Read on to find out how the four seasons of beauty foods support your changing beauty needs, from spring detox to winter dryness.

BANANA BUCKWHEAT PANCAKES

Pancakes are a weekend treat, but your average syrup-coated breakfast flapjacks put you in a blood sugar slump and leave your skin prone to breakouts. This antiaging pancake recipe swaps white flour and refined sugar for mineral-rich buckwheat flour and low glycemic maple syrup. The banana lends its own sweetness, so you can even skip the syrup. Toss a few finely chopped walnuts into the batter for crunch and extra antiaging omega-3s.

Serves 2 to 4

1 cup/240 ml unsweetened
  almond milk
4 tsp white vinegar
1 cup/115 g buckwheat flour
½ tsp sea salt
½ tsp baking powder
¼ tsp baking soda

¼ cup/25 g raw walnut halves,
  finely chopped (optional)
1 ripe banana
2 tbsp pure maple syrup
1½ tbsp organic butter or coconut
  oil, melted, plus more for frying
1 egg

Combine the almond milk and vinegar in a mug and set aside for 5 minutes. In a medium bowl, whisk together the flour, salt, baking powder, baking soda, and walnuts, if using. In another medium bowl, mash the banana with a fork. Mix in the maple syrup, melted butter, egg, and the almond milk mixture. Pour the liquid ingredients into the dry ingredients and stir briefly to incorporate. Heat a greased skillet to medium heat. Drop the batter in ¼-cup/60-ml measures into the hot pan. After small bubbles form on top, about 60 seconds, flip the pancakes and cook the other side for about 30 seconds. Transfer to a plate and keep warm while you cook the remaining pancakes. Re-grease the pan as needed to prevent sticking. Serve warm.

OMEGA BEAUTY BITES

Why is it that some of the smelliest foods (onions, garlic, and, yes, sardines) are so beautifying? You might not want to tote a sardine-packed lunch to the office, but whipping up these omega-3 and protein-rich bites for breakfast provides supercharged fuel to start your day. The bite-sized pieces are perfect to pop in your mouth as you get ready to leave the house for the day—just remember to brush afterward.

Serves 2 to 3

Two 4-oz/125-g tins skinless and
  boneless water-packed sardines,
  drained
2 tbsp vegan natural mayonnaise
⅛ tsp ground turmeric

⅛ tsp ground black pepper
2 tbsp minced fresh parsley
½ organic cucumber
3 sheets nori

In a medium bowl, mash the sardines with a fork. Mix in the mayonnaise, turmeric, pepper, and parsley. Cut twelve 4-in/ 10-cm matchsticks from your cucumber half and set them aside. Finely mince the rest of the cucumber half and add to the sardine mixture. Place the nori sheets on a work surface, shiny side down. Beginning about 1 in/2.5 cm from the edge nearest to you, spread one-third of the sardine mixture over each sheet, leaving about 2 in/5 cm bare on the opposite end. Place 4 of the cucumber matchsticks lengthwise across the sardine mixture at the near edge of each nori sheet and, again starting from the edge near you, roll tightly into a sushi-esque roll. Seal each roll by wetting the seam and pressing down firmly. Using a sharp knife, cut each nori roll into six 1-in/2.5-cm pieces, trimming off messy ends, if needed, and serve.

OATMEAL-RAISIN COOKIE TRUFFLES

These truffles are the perfect beautifying antidote to a sugar craving. They're sweetened with raisins, and are full of antioxidant-rich spices and beauty minerals.

Makes 12 truffles

1 cup/100 g raw walnuts
½ cup/85 g raisins
¼ cup/20 g gluten-free whole oats
½ tsp ground cinnamon
⅛ tsp ground cloves

⅛ tsp sea salt
4 tsp unsweetened almond milk
Unsweetened shredded coconut
 for coating

In a food processor, combine the walnuts, raisins, and oats and pulse just until a coarse meal forms. Transfer to a medium bowl. Add the cinnamon, cloves, and salt and stir to combine. Stir in the almond milk. Using the back of a spoon, mash until the mixture leaves the sides of the bowl and forms one large clump. Pour a deep layer of shredded coconut onto a plate. Pinch off pieces of the truffle dough and shape into 1-in/2.5-cm balls. Roll in the shredded coconut to coat and chill for 10 to 15 minutes before serving.

MAPLE SESAME MILLET

This savory-sweet breakfast dish was inspired by a candy I encountered in London. While that sugary treat wasn't skin-friendly, this recipe is, thanks to maple syrup, which has a lower glycemic index than sugar, and a foundation of protein- and fiber-packed millet to promote steady blood sugar. Feel free to substitute another Eat Pretty grain, like quinoa or gluten-free oats.

Serves 2

½ cup/100 g dried millet, rinsed
  and drained
1½ cups/360 ml water
Sea salt

2 tbsp tahini
2 tbsp unsweetened almond milk
2 tsp pure maple syrup or raw
  honey

Combine the millet and water in a saucepan and add a pinch of salt. Bring to a boil over high heat, then reduce the heat to medium-low and simmer, uncovered, for about 15 minutes, or until the millet is tender. Remove from the heat and drain any excess water. Stir in the tahini. Divide between two bowls and top each portion with 1 tbsp almond milk and 1 tsp maple syrup. Serve warm.

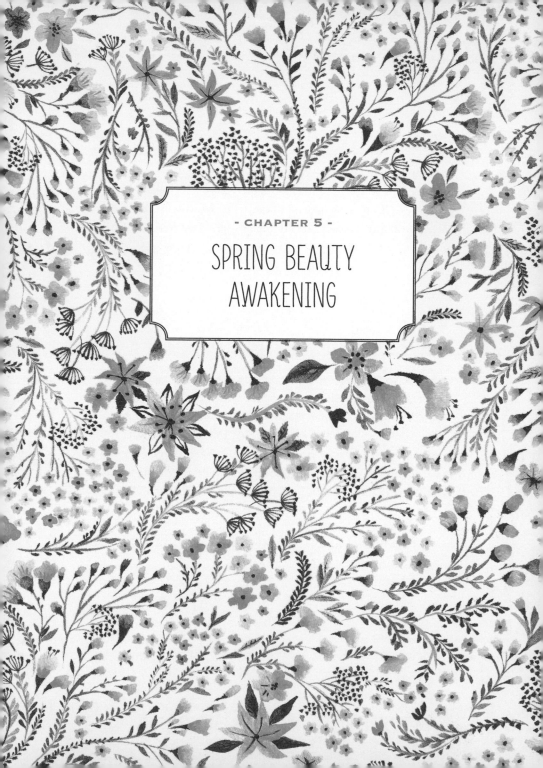

- CHAPTER 5 -

SPRING BEAUTY
AWAKENING

If you're reading Eat Pretty for the first time, it may feel like your own personal spring; it's your moment of reinvention. If it's not actually springtime in your part of the world, you'll still want to read through each of the following seasonal chapters, then return to focus on the beauty foods and beauty needs of your particular season. And wherever you are in your beauty and wellness journey, you can use the energy and possibility of spring to inspire you. What do you want to see in the mirror? How do you want to feel? What do you want your relationship with food to look like? Embrace the possibility that awaits you, this spring and for as long as you lead the Eat Pretty life.

If spring is here on your calendar, that means you made it through another long winter! It's the moment to celebrate the rebirth of beauty that happens year after year in nature, and this year we're also celebrating you. This spring, as you watch barren twigs push forth tender buds that sprout into glossy green leaves, think of your own blossoming. When was the last time you pushed yourself forward to create a beautiful bloom? A commitment to Eat Pretty is your opportunity. This spring is your season to come alive again—to regain your energy, your radiance, and find yourself renewed.

In Eastern teachings, every season connects to two or three organs of the body that particularly require our support as they work hard to meet our seasonal needs for beauty and health. Spring is our season for detoxification, and the liver and the gallbladder, two essential detoxifying organs, are the organs we will support in the months ahead. This doesn't require extra work on your part, because you'll already find an abundance of beauty foods to support liver and gallbladder health in the spring harvest. All you need to do is eat spring beauty foods.

Detox is a natural function that your body performs every day, but it's most effective when you support it with beauty foods and healthy habits. Which brings me to a special note on an increasingly popular ritual: the juice fast. Don't get too starry-eyed about formal cleanse and detox programs—especially juice-only versions—without applying what you've already learned in *Eat Pretty*. All juices (and detoxes) are not created equal—some are incredibly nutritious, while others are sugar bombs that leave you feeling sluggish, cloudy-headed, and ravenous. Juices are often very low in fiber and very high in sugar (about the same amount that you'd get in a can of soda), so they spike your blood sugar quickly and leave you in a slump. They can even contribute to wrinkles and breakouts. The health and beauty benefits of juice depend very much on its particular ingredients. A no-brainer, right? Just because your detox comes in a liquid form and includes some beauty foods does not mean that it will make your skin and body happy.

Spring is the season of shedding—pounds, clutter, Beauty Betrayer foods, old habits—to make room for new beauty. Not only should you spring-clean your beauty routine and toss out old makeup, toxic products, even colors that you've just been wearing for too long, you should cleanse your cabinets of food that isn't supportive of your beauty and health. In the spirit of renewal that comes with spring, you'll want to freshen your look and update your wardrobe to reflect the radiant new you. The green of spring signals planning, growth, development, inspired action, and ambition—let those feelings characterize this season in your life.

It's time to get excited that your body is growing healthier and more beautiful every day. Reinforce the commitment you've made to nourish your beauty by trying new products this spring. Make them natural or organic, to support your hormone health and lighten the toxic burden on your body. If you're not sure where to start, try scent: find a perfume to suit your springtime mood, one that doesn't contain synthetic fragrance and hormone-disrupting phthalates. (See my picks in the Resources section on page 200.)

This chapter and the three following it unfold the season-by-season plans I created to help you move mindfully, energetically, and, of course, beautifully through the year. The spring plan starts with a list of beauty intentions that describe the most powerful changes you can make for your beauty and body this spring. Then you'll explore the most beautifying ways to eat during the spring, complete with detailed info about the freshest seasonal foods that help you glow from the inside out. You'll find simple recipes to help you incorporate those foods into your diet right away. Remember that you plant the seeds for abundant beauty with every small change you make. The seeds that you plant this spring will sprout and bloom vibrantly in the seasons ahead.

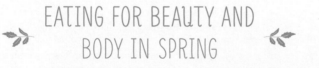

☙ BEAUTY EDITOR NOTE ❧

This spring, add Epsom salts to your bath to increase your body's natural detox abilities and boost your intake of calming magnesium.

EATING FOR BEAUTY AND BODY IN SPRING

Welcoming spring doesn't just mean trading sweaters for T-shirts and choosing brighter nail polish colors—there are deeper ways to spring-ify your looks! Start by going green. Hit the farmers' market and fill up on chlorophyll-rich green foods that help you detox, oxygenate your blood, and shed pounds this season. Think of spring greens as your edible beauty tonic. It's amazing to see just how many spring beauty foods naturally support detox and liver and gallbladder health, reduce water retention, and increase antiaging glutathione in our bodies. The earth seems to be helping us out of our long season of rest, into a period of youthfulness and energy. It truly is a season of renewal for our body and our beauty. In order to achieve the most gorgeous transformation, make

Your SPRING Beauty Intentions

Starting a new season with a focus on your beauty intentions for the months ahead gives you a clear course toward your beauty and health goals. Keep a copy of this list where you can refer to it all season long to turn these short-term goals into long-term beauty habits.

1. **Fill up on cleansing fluids.** Boost your body's natural detox abilities by drinking pure filtered water or a beverage with additional liver-supporting properties, like lemon water or dandelion root tea. Juice or blend green veggies and herbs like celery, kale, and parsley into a chlorophyll-rich detox drink, or sip filtered hot water throughout the day.

2. **Plant seeds.** Connect with the earth this season by bringing fresh flowers and plants into your home, and growing food or flowers to enjoy in the months ahead. Watching seeds sprout and develop into nourishing beauty foods come summer can be a deeply grounding experience.

3. **Lighten up your liver.** The liver is one of the main blood purifiers in the body. Liver sluggishness can manifest in skin issues like acne and eczema, and in allergies to food and environment. Show your liver some daily love with morning lemon water, and by packing your diet full of chlorophyll-rich, alkaline green foods like asparagus, spinach, and sprouts.

4. **Simplify supper.** The delicate foods of spring retain their valuable beauty nutrients when they're lightly steamed or eaten raw. Avoid browning or burning your foods and you'll also prevent AGE formation in the body. Try no-fuss cooking methods like blanching or sautéing with water or vegetable broth to save calories and ease the digestive burden on your body.

5. **Reduce toxins.** All toxins, whether they come from food, prescription drugs, personal care products, or our environment, overload our liver with filtering duties. Reducing your consumption of processed and pesticide-laden foods is one of the most effective ways to detox and support your beauty this season—and year-round.

sure your food choices reflect energy and life. Instead of aluminum cans and plastic packages, choose bunches of greens, cartons of strawberries, and handfuls of fresh herbs.

This spring, commit to a morning ritual that you'll continue all year long: a glass of warm lemon water first thing in the morning to prepare your digestive system for the day ahead, support a well-functioning liver, and nourish incredibly radiant skin. Smoothies make appealing spring breakfasts (try my Lemony Beauty Smoothie on page 94), since they're light, and ideal vehicles for greens and veggies that energize your cells. Spirulina, hemp, and pea protein powder make great sources of vegetarian protein to add to smoothies. For convenience purposes, green smoothies are as portable as a muffin or pastry—and so much more beautifying.

Mid-morning, follow your smoothie with a healthy snack. Try a handful of nuts, a banana with almond butter, or naturally smoked wild salmon and avocado—a combination of protein and healthy fats. You may find that your appetite diminishes a bit this season, so your spring lunches are likely to be light, like soups (it's still chilly out!), salads, or lettuce and nori wraps. Again, make sure your meals contain blood sugar–stabilizing protein or complex carbs, whether they come from a grain like quinoa or an animal source like pastured eggs or sardines, as well as healthy fats to help you absorb the nutrients from your veggie-based meals.

Bitter greens like endive and dandelion are especially cleansing to the body, even in small amounts, so spice up salads and wraps with a handful. To help build healthy gut bacteria that will efficiently break down and assimilate nutrients from these fresh, raw foods, try to eat cultured veggies once a day—a brined pickle, a few forkfuls of kimchi, or a glass of kefir will do the trick.

Use your evening meal as an opportunity to try out some new Eat Pretty foods (remember, simple is beautiful, so don't feel the stress to create a perfect plate). Quinoa, asparagus, greens, wild salmon, and pastured eggs are some of my favorite foundations for spring suppers.

For sweetness, fill up on ripe berries and the remaining citrus of the season, but otherwise make a big effort to reduce sugar. Treat yourself to a few chocolate eggs or a traditional dessert that's special to you during the spring holidays, but go for a less-is-more approach to sugar. Less sugar, more gorgeous. Come summer, you'll be ready to show a little more skin.

The Eat Pretty
➤➤ SPRING BEAUTY BASKET ⬅⬅

It's the season to reinvent your beauty, Eat Pretty–style. Spring beauty foods are fresh, green, light, and packed with natural detox abilities. Celebrate the newness of the season by filling your diet with these crisp greens, spicy bulbs, aromatic herbs, tender shoots, and juicy berries, all of which will restore youth and energy to your beauty and body in the months ahead. For more information on the beauty nutrients in these foods, refer to the Beauty Nutrients chart (page 46) and the Phytochemical Beauty Boosters chart (page 51).

ARTICHOKE: Slow Beauty

Peeling away the leaves of an artichoke bite by bite is a lovely way to savor its fresh, spring beauty and anticipate its decadent, nutrient-packed heart. The artichoke is an ideal spring beauty veggie. Its high fiber makes it a highly cleansing food, as does its phytochemical silymarin, which supports both liver and gallbladder health. Artichokes stimulate bile production in the liver, aiding in detox and the digestion of fats. They're a diuretic food that prevents bloating and eases digestion all-around, making them a recommended food for tummy troubles like irritable bowel syndrome (IBS). As a beauty food, they rank high for their support of healthy levels of glutathione, an extremely powerful antiaging nutrient.

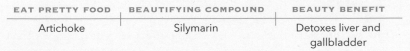

EAT PRETTY FOOD	BEAUTIFYING COMPOUND	BEAUTY BENEFIT
Artichoke	Silymarin	Detoxes liver and gallbladder

ARUGULA: Spicy, Sexy Green

Here's an easy way to rev up your antiaging capacity and your digestion at the same time: eat arugula. The sulfur-containing glucosinolates in arugula, when chopped or chewed, release other phytochemicals that lower inflammation, protect cells from DNA damage, reduce skin redness caused by the sun, and defend against UV damage. This powerful protection extends for several days after eating! Arugula is rich in vitamin K for strong bones and fewer dark circles, and it's packed with chlorophyll. Peppery arugula is also a detox booster; add some to spring salads to celebrate this season of cleansing.

EAT PRETTY FOOD	BEAUTIFYING COMPOUND	BEAUTY BENEFIT
Arugula	Glucosinolates	Protect cells from DNA damage

ASPARAGUS: Glutathione Booster

These slender spring veggies are more powerful than they look, with about 15 percent of your daily iron in just a few stalks. Asparagus is one of the best foods in the world for folate, a B vitamin that is important for DNA synthesis and cell repair. For beauty, the glutathione levels in asparagus are especially exciting, since glutathione is one of the most powerful antioxidant defenders in our antiaging diet. Glutathione is a special protector of our mitochondria, which increase the energy and oxygen-carrying capacity of our blood. Glutathione levels decline with age (starting as early as thirty!), so we need to eat as many glutathione-boosting foods as we can to look and feel youthful and radiant. This spring, eat asparagus raw or lightly steamed (dip it in tasty hummus) for the highest glutathione levels.

EAT PRETTY FOOD	BEAUTIFYING COMPOUND	BEAUTY BENEFIT
Asparagus	Glutathione	Powerful antioxidant

COCONUT: *Tropical Beauty Treat*

A natural powerhouse, coconut brims with beauty benefits, from oil to water to meat. Coconut water is a fantastic fluid for electrolyte, or mineral, balance (far better than a sports drink), since it contains potassium, magnesium, and sodium, plus small amounts of zinc, copper, and selenium. Proper electrolyte balance means that your heart delivers oxygenated blood efficiently throughout your body, setting your skin aglow. Selenium is an important antiaging mineral that maintains skin elasticity and a healthy scalp, while zinc keeps hair and nails gorgeous and immunity strong. On a day when you're looking and feeling just a bit lackluster, treat yourself to a young coconut for a special beauty elixir. You can distinguish young coconuts from the common, dark brown variety by their white husks and cylindrical shape with a pointed top.

EAT PRETTY FOOD	BEAUTIFYING COMPOUND	BEAUTY BENEFIT
Coconut	Potassium	Supports healthy electrolyte balance

DANDELION GREENS: *From Weed to Superfood*

Chowing down on greens that are traditionally seen as weeds may seem odd to some, but in-the-know beauties will attest to the major detox benefits of dandelion greens. Want clearer, brighter skin? Dandelion is traditionally used as an acne and eczema remedy. Some of its skin benefits come from its liver and kidney support and overall digestive boosting abilities. Additional benefits come from its content of vitamin A; a handful of dandelion greens has over 100 percent of your daily vitamin A needs. Dandelion greens also have diuretic properties that reduce bloating. Dandelion greens are bitter, so I suggest tossing a handful into a green smoothie, or mixing them up with other greens in a salad. That bitter flavor is a reminder of their cleansing properties! For another way to enjoy the beauty benefits of dandelion, check out earthy dandelion root tea.

EAT PRETTY FOOD	BEAUTIFYING COMPOUND	BEAUTY BENEFIT
Dandelion greens	Vitamin A	Keeps skin clear and glowing

ENDIVE: 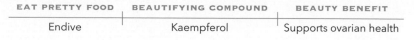Ovary Protector

One small head of this crunchy, mildly bitter type of chicory provides twice your daily needs for skin-smoothing vitamin A, which could explain its traditional use as an acne tonic. Its role in liver detox and bile production also makes it a major boon to a clear, gorgeous complexion. Endive is a mild laxative that's excellent for digestion. It also promotes overall health of the ovaries: eating endive has been shown to help reduce the risk of many types of cancer, including breast, lung, and ovarian, thanks to a detoxifying phytochemical called kaempferol. With a water content of over 90 percent, endive is very low in calories relative to the powerful dose of beauty nutrition you'll get in every bite.

EAT PRETTY FOOD	BEAUTIFYING COMPOUND	BEAUTY BENEFIT
Endive	Kaempferol	Supports ovarian health

GARLIC: 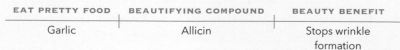Ward off Colds—and Wrinkles

Garlic is off the charts for its anti-inflammatory value, exactly what you want for preventing disease (including cancer) and quelling beauty issues like acne and skin sensitivity. Allicin, a sulfurous phytochemical that gives garlic its distinctive taste and smell, fights off signs of aging by protecting a powerful enzyme that stops the action of other collagen-digesting enzymes in the body. Garlic, with its antibacterial and antifungal properties, supports your healthy intestinal flora, which is vitally important for the absorption of beautifying nutrients. Garlic boosts circulation, and supports the production of detoxifying glutathione in the body, keeping your antiaging defenses in top form. To get the most from every garlic clove, let it sit for about 15 minutes after crushing or chopping to allow its powerful compounds to activate.

EAT PRETTY FOOD	BEAUTIFYING COMPOUND	BEAUTY BENEFIT
Garlic	Allicin	Stops wrinkle formation

GREEN BEANS: The Skinny on Elasticity

Green beans, or string beans, are sources of highly absorbable silicon, which strengthens connective tissue and keeps your skin, hair, and nails flexible and strong. These anti-inflammatory veggies also contain an impressive range of antiaging phytochemicals, from sun-protective carotenoids and quercetin to free radical–fighting catechins. They're good sources of hair- and nail-building minerals like iron, thiamine, riboflavin, and niacin, as well as manganese, an important nutrient for building bones and connective tissue.

EAT PRETTY FOOD	BEAUTIFYING COMPOUND	BEAUTY BENEFIT
Green beans	Silicon	Promotes skin strength and elasticity

LEMON: Daily Detox

If you're an Eat Pretty eater, lemons are one fruit that you'll always have in your kitchen. They're said to be freshest and best tasting in early spring, a season when your body craves the powerful alkaline detoxification boost that their juice provides. You probably know that lemons are chock-full of collagen-building vitamin C, but they're also rich in immune-boosting bioflavonoids (found in highest concentration in the pith and rind). Bioflavonoids boost lymph flow and strengthen blood vessels, aiding in the prevention of varicose veins. Lemons are liver-loving beauty foods with astringent properties that clean out the digestive tract, stimulate bile and saliva, and cleanse the blood. Lemons also have diuretic and laxative effects, so they help you maintain a flat belly all day.

> ❧ BEAUTY EDITOR NOTE ❧
>
> *Lemon peels contain alpha-hydroxy acids that tighten, brighten, and exfoliate. Rub a fresh peel gently on dark spots, rough patches, or stained nails to lighten and smooth, then rinse with cool water.*

EAT PRETTY FOOD	BEAUTIFYING COMPOUND	BEAUTY BENEFIT
Lemon	Bioflavonoids	Strengthen blood vessels

PEAS: Protein Booster

Protein is essential for strong hair, nails, and collagen, and peas happen to be an amazing source of veggie protein (about 10 g in a small bowl). The protein and fiber in peas keep blood sugar steady, while their phytochemicals prevent DNA damage and boost immunity. Peas are a great source of B vitamins, especially thiamine, which your body needs for healthy nervous system function, and folate, for cell repair. Spring peas are sweet and crisp, so try them raw!

EAT PRETTY FOOD	BEAUTIFYING COMPOUND	BEAUTY BENEFIT
Peas	Vitamin B₁/ thiamine	Supports nervous system function and digestion

RADISH: Spicy Nail Booster

These crisp, spicy members of the mustard family are triple threats against wrinkled, lackluster skin. They are a fantastic veggie source of vitamin C, as well as a source of the rare but essential beauty minerals sulfur and silicon to nourish healthy, supple, glowing skin and strong connective tissue, including gorgeous nails. Crunching away at these beauties helps reduce water retention, ease digestion, and clean out stagnation, thanks to their peppery bite and their liver- and kidney-supporting properties. They're also known to support thyroid health and balance. With few calories (just 20 or so in a large handful), you'll want to add radishes to your Eat Pretty diet as often as possible this spring.

EAT PRETTY FOOD	BEAUTIFYING COMPOUND	BEAUTY BENEFIT
Radish	Silicon	Builds strong bone and connective tissue

RHUBARB: Sweet without the Sugar

Joining the ranks of spring's powerfully detoxifying harvest is rhubarb, a veggie (not a fruit!) with phytochemicals like lycopene and quercetin to protect your skin from sun damage. The astringent nature of rhubarb makes it a cooling, detoxifying food that supports liver health and strong digestion. Rhubarb is an excellent source of calcium, with over 10 percent of your daily calcium in a good-size stalk or two. Just don't eat it stewed in sugar syrup, as in a pie filling; try chopped rhubarb roasted with a little salt and coconut oil for salads or in a savory tart.

EAT PRETTY FOOD	BEAUTIFYING COMPOUND	BEAUTY BENEFIT
Rhubarb	Lycopene	Defends against sun damage

ROMAINE LETTUCE: More Beauty Bang for Your Buck

Lettuce may be super-light on calories, but its nutrients make it a beauty heavyweight. One packed handful of romaine lettuce (a mere 8 calories) provides more than 80 percent of your daily vitamin A needs. That means a helping of romaine salad keeps your skin smooth, youthful, and supple for yet another day. Romaine lettuce is a good source of folate, for healthy cell repair, and silicon, for strong hair, nails, and skin. If you don't have time to make (or chew) a salad, blend a whole head of romaine into your green smoothies (you'll only add about 100 calories) to deliver one-third of your daily iron, 8 g of protein, and a major dose of B vitamins and beauty minerals. Talk about bang for your buck!

EAT PRETTY FOOD	BEAUTIFYING COMPOUND	BEAUTY BENEFIT
Romaine lettuce	Vitamin A	Supports smooth skin

SPINACH: Powerful Green Beauty

Eating spinach boosts levels of two major antiaging nutrients: vitamin A and glutathione. Eat Pretty eaters want both in their beauty routines! Vitamin A keeps skin-cell turnover humming along, making your complexion glowy, while glutathione defends against DNA and mitochondrial damage and regenerates vitamin C for extended antioxidant power. Spinach is highly nourishing to the eyes and the liver, and it contains compounds that protect the lining of the digestive tract from inflammation. It's also bursting with blood-oxygenating chlorophyll and beauty minerals like iron, manganese, and magnesium. And forget the milk—spinach has a major dose of bone-strengthening vitamin K. While raw spinach is a major beauty food, the calcium and eye-protective lutein content in its leaves is more easily absorbed when it is cooked. Eat spinach with vitamin C–rich foods like lemon or strawberries to aid in the absorption of its beauty nutrients.

EAT PRETTY FOOD	BEAUTIFYING COMPOUND	BEAUTY BENEFIT
Spinach	Vitamin A	Supports cell renewal and repair

SPROUTS: *Living Beauty Nutrition*

Sprouted seeds and beans come in many varieties, each generally packed with more vitamins, protein, and healthy fats than their unsprouted relatives. Sprouts are full of enzymes, making them easily digestible sources of antiaging nutrients that help you get the most beauty from every bite. Our natural enzyme production decreases with age, so taking in enzymes from living, sprouted food helps improve digestion and keep our bodies young. When you sprout seeds or beans, they come alive with nutrition. Broccoli sprouts specifically are a powerful source of antiaging, glutathione-boosting sulforaphane, but other sprouts like mung beans and radish seeds are mighty beauty foods, too. (The flours and grains you see in the store in bags and baked goods labeled "sprouted" were indeed sprouted before drying or milling to increase digestibility and bioavailability of some nutrients, but they're not living, growing products.)

EAT PRETTY FOOD	BEAUTIFYING COMPOUND	BEAUTY BENEFIT
Sprouts	Enzymes	Boost nutrient absorption

STRAWBERRIES: 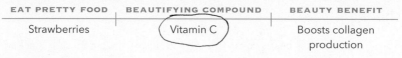 Sweet Cs

Fruit is scarce in the spring, so juicy strawberries steal the show with their sweetness. These anti-inflammatory berries increase the antioxidant capacity of your blood, defending you from stress and signs of aging. Eat them for their collagen-building, free radical–fighting vitamin C (one handful of strawberries has even more C than a whole orange) that also boosts metabolism and increases fat burning. They also contain manganese, which supports mitochondrial defense. Among their many antiaging phytochemicals, ellagic acid in strawberries aids in blood sugar balance and helps maintain healthy, youthful cells.

EAT PRETTY FOOD	BEAUTIFYING COMPOUND	BEAUTY BENEFIT
Strawberries	Vitamin C	Boosts collagen production

SUGAR SNAP PEAS: 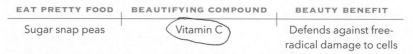 Crispy and Crave-Worthy

This crispy veggie is slightly sweet, with an edible pod. It looks similar to a shelling pea, but here the fresh, crunchy pod is its main draw. One handful of sugar snap peas contains a dose of protein—though at about 3 g, not quite as much as shelling peas—and plenty of collagen-building vitamin C (about 98 percent of your daily needs!) and iron, making sugar snap peas an excellent booster for hair, skin, and nails alike. And with only about 40 calories in a 1-cup/140-g serving, you can indulge your sweet cravings all spring long.

EAT PRETTY FOOD	BEAUTIFYING COMPOUND	BEAUTY BENEFIT
Sugar snap peas	Vitamin C	Defends against free-radical damage to cells

WATERCRESS: DNA Rescuer

This super-charged cruciferous veggie not only packs in a load of beautifying nutrients, it's also powerful enough to repair DNA damage. One of watercress's antiaging phytochemicals, sulforaphane, defends against free-radical damage to DNA, reduces redness caused by sun exposure, lowers inflammation, and boosts glutathione production. The wealth of beauty vitamins (A, C, K) in watercress keeps skin, hair, nails, and vision healthy and helps prevent future damage there, too. The diuretic properties of watercress also make it an effective natural detox, so it's ideal to blend into green smoothies.

EAT PRETTY FOOD	BEAUTIFYING COMPOUND	BEAUTY BENEFIT
Watercress	Sulforaphane	Defends against DNA damage

SPRING AT A GLANCE

You now have the tools to remake your beauty, cell by cell, this spring! At this moment, you haven't even begun to imagine how gorgeous you will look and feel when you feed your beauty from the inside out, and you won't know until you get started. Fill this spring with the foods, meals, thoughts, and habits that pamper and support your body and you'll start an incredible transformation that lasts for seasons—and years—to come.

LEMONY BEAUTY SMOOTHIE

Switch up this smoothie throughout the year by substituting fresh, seasonal greens. Throw in some basil or mint in the summer, or kale in the fall. I like to add a small amount of organic lemon peel for flavor and extra bioflavonoids.

Serves 2 to 4

2 cups/480 ml water
2 large handfuls of spinach leaves
1 medium handful of dandelion
  greens or watercress
1 medium handful of parsley, thick
  stems removed

½ ripe avocado
1 organic lemon, peeled
½ frozen banana (use the whole
  banana if you prefer more
  sweetness)

In a high-powered blender, combine the water, spinach, dandelion greens, and parsley, and blend to a coarse purée. Add the avocado, lemon (and some strips of the peel, if you like), and banana. Blend on high until smooth and creamy. Serve immediately.

QUINOA ASPARAGUS PILAF

This detoxifying spring dish boosts glutathione levels in the body, for all-over antiaging benefits. If you prefer, you can prepare the pilaf in advance and serve at room temperature.

Serves 4 to 6

1 tsp coconut oil
2 shallots, finely chopped
1 bunch fresh chives, chopped
  into ½-in/12-mm pieces
1½ cups/260 g quinoa, rinsed and
  drained

1½ cups/360 ml vegetable broth
1 bunch slender asparagus, cut
  into 1½-in/4-cm pieces
Juice of 1 lemon

In a large sauté pan, melt the coconut oil over medium heat. Add the shallots and cook until they begin to soften, about 5 minutes. Add half of the chives and cook for 2 minutes longer. Add the quinoa and broth, raise the heat to high, and bring to a boil. Reduce the heat to maintain a simmer, cover, and cook for 10 minutes. Uncover, add the asparagus and lemon juice, and stir to combine. Re-cover and cook until the liquid is absorbed, about 10 minutes longer. Remove from the heat and let stand for 5 minutes. Top with the remaining chives and serve.

RAINBOW TROUT WITH WATERCRESS PESTO

This nutty, sharp pesto pairs perfectly with mellow, flaky trout. Make a double batch of pesto and toss it with pasta or spread it over sandwiches—it's as versatile as traditional basil pesto, with even bigger antiaging benefits.

Serves 2

2 fillets rainbow trout, 4 to 6 oz/
   115 to 170 g each
1 tsp organic unsalted butter
1 bunch watercress
2 tbsp olive oil

2 tbsp pine nuts
1 tbsp nutritional yeast
Sea salt and freshly ground
   black pepper

Preheat the broiler.

Rinse the trout fillets, pat dry, and place, skin-side down, on a baking sheet lined with greased aluminum foil. Melt the butter and brush over the fillets. Set aside.

In a food processor, combine the watercress (leaves and stems) and olive oil and pulse until the cress is finely chopped but not liquefied. Add the pine nuts and nutritional yeast and pulse until combined. Season with salt and pepper. Spread a thick layer of the pesto over each fillet. Place the pan under the broiler and broil until the fish is sizzling and the pesto just begins to brown on top, about 5 minutes. Serve hot.

CREAMY STRAWBERRY ALMOND TART

I love this decadent spring dessert for special occasions—you'd never guess that the creamy texture comes from cashews, not dairy!

Serves 10 to 12

CRUST:
1½ cups/130 g almond meal
¼ cup/45 g bittersweet chocolate chunks (at least 70 percent cocoa)
⅔ cup/110 g pitted dates
¼ tsp sea salt
¼ tsp ground cinnamon

FILLING:
2½ cups/225 g raw cashews, soaked in water for 4 hours
2½ cups/280 g strawberries
⅔ cup/150 g coconut oil, melted
¼ cup/60 ml pure maple syrup
3 drops liquid stevia
½ tsp almond extract
Scant ½ tsp sea salt

To make the crust: In a food processor, combine the almond meal, chocolate, dates, salt, and cinnamon and pulse until coarsely combined. Line a 9-in/23-cm cake pan with wax paper, leaving an overhang of the paper on either side that will allow you to lift up the tart later. Press the crust mixture firmly into the bottom and up the sides of the lined pan and keep cool in the freezer while you prep the filling.

To make the filling: Drain and rinse the soaked cashews. In a food processor, combine the cashews, strawberries, melted coconut oil, maple syrup, and stevia and process to a coarse purée. Add the almond extract and salt and process until completely smooth.

Pour the filling into the chilled crust. Return the tart to the freezer until well chilled and firm, at least 3 hours or overnight.

To unmold the tart, run a hot knife around the edge and use the wax paper to lift and transfer to a serving dish. Thaw for at least 2 hours in the refrigerator before cutting into wedges and serving.

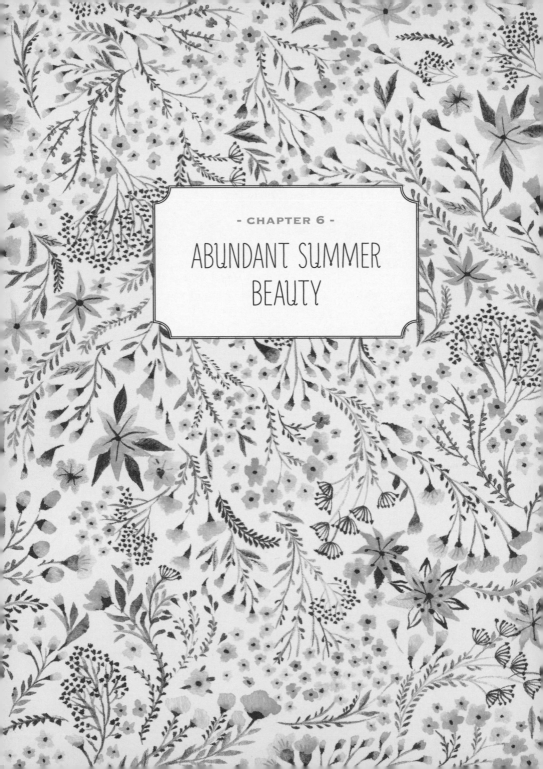

- CHAPTER 6 -

ABUNDANT SUMMER BEAUTY

If spring was your season to plant the seeds of beauty, summer is your radiance in full bloom. If you chose an abundance of detoxifying Eat Pretty foods during the spring, you're already looking and feeling incredible. With the arrival of summer sunshine, you'll experience even more of the energy and glow that you've been anticipating since you started building your lifestyle of beauty. Summer is the season of abundant beauty, and you have it to spare this year!

I have exciting goals for you in the season ahead. I want you to use Eat Pretty foods to sustain your beauty and body and help defend it from the aging UV rays of the sun. I want your skin to be so deeply nourished that you feel radiant without makeup on hot summer days. I want you to sweat and shine free of melting foundation, and feel confident that you look more beautiful than ever before. There's something different about you now that you've embraced Eat Pretty practices. You can already feel it, can't you?

Summer beauty is not just alive; it's lush and thriving. The beauty of nature is everywhere—in the air, the trees, and on your seasonal plate. Great skin is your best accessory this season, and sometimes you'll be showing a whole lot of it. Experiment with head-turning pops of color in your wardrobe and in your makeup, or try a highlighter on your cheekbones and brow bone to give a dewy, youthful luminosity to your skin. It feels less risky to get noticed when you're confident about your skin and your body, so embrace the spotlight.

Summer is also the season of creativity and activity, and you should feel inspired, energetic, and full of intention to continue your lifestyle of beauty. If you need a little help, again, look around at nature. Even if you're still on a journey to be your best self (and we all are), live in the moment this summer. Don't skip the chance to plunge into the ocean because you don't yet have the bikini body you want, and don't opt out of a barbecue because you don't want to face a table full of Beauty Betrayer foods. Make your own beautifying dish and share the benefits. The Blueberry Lentil Salad on page 115 and the Green Wraps with Tilapia, Pineapple, Cucumber, and Sun-Dried Tomato Pesto on page 117 are perfect for picnics. Remember how profoundly your personal happiness influences your head-to-toe glow. When you're feeling great thanks to mood-boosting beauty foods and stable blood sugar, and glowing from within—you'll get a natural bronze from summer foods' skin-tinting carotenoids—you're not the only one who notices the radiant you.

Depending on where you live, summer might be hot and dry or hot and humid; either way you'll battle sun damage. To maintain a summer glow without risking redness and future wrinkles, your best weapons are both a broad-spectrum natural sunscreen and an anti-inflammatory, UV-protective beauty diet packed with the foods in this chapter. Sunscreen doesn't always play nice with blemish-prone skin, so look for a natural sunscreen formula that feels light on your skin. Twice a week, or as needed, use a lightly exfoliating mask or a soft washcloth to remove any stubborn sunscreen that's building up. Always be gentle; you don't want to scrub so enthusiastically that you sensitize your skin and strip away its natural barrier, which is essential for environmental defense. Of course, you'll also be eating antiacne foods and skipping Beauty Betrayers this season, and that makes clear skin much easier to maintain even when you throw sunscreen into the mix.

If you've let your exercise routine lag, or you just can't find workout motivation, this is your season to bring the beauty of movement into your life. Wake up with the sun and jog or bike before the sun is hottest. Take advantage of the extended daylight with an evening walk, and use that walk as an opportunity to practice walking meditation (yes, it counts as meditation, too!). As you walk, let your thoughts rest on your breath and steps alone, not your to-do list.

🍃 BEAUTY EDITOR NOTE 🍃

Chilled green tea can be a healing, redness-relieving toner or face mist for sun-damaged skin. Just use your brew within a day or two of steeping for the maximum skin benefits.

Travel, too, adds to the movement and energy of summer. You might be jet-setting solo to chic destinations, or hauling a car full of kids to the beach. It's all about playing, and creating meaningful experiences that will keep you glowing when winter

rolls back around. This is a physically beautiful time of the year; experience it to its fullest. Turn down the frigid air conditioning and feel the warmth of the season in your body (though you might need cooler temps for sleeping). Dig your hands in the dirt and watch a flower bloom under your care. This is summer beauty to savor.

Summer is the season to support the heart and the small intestine. The heart is the major circulator of beauty nutrition within our bodies. The small intestine assimilates nutrition from the beauty foods we consume, linking it closely to the appearance of our skin, hair, and nails and the overall health of our body. This is the season to care for these two critical organs that help us absorb and circulate beauty nutrition and maintain boundless summer energy.

Every day is a new chance to feed your beauty, and every small choice contributes to major change. If you made it through the spring with Eat Pretty changes to your lifestyle, celebrate the solstice and the deepening beauty that is yours this summer. Ahead, you'll find your seasonal intentions and the top high-season beauty foods and recipes to nourish your beauty from the inside.

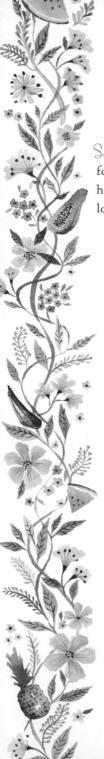

Your SUMMER Beauty Intentions

Starting a new season with a focus on your beauty intentions for the months ahead gives you a clear course toward your beauty and health goals. Keep a copy of this list where you can refer to it all season long to turn these short-term goals into long-term beauty habits.

1. Eat pretty—and cool. Water-rich beauty foods like watermelon, cantaloupe, cucumber, celery, watercress, lemons, and coconut water keep your body cool when it's sweltering outdoors. They're also natural diuretics, so you'll be slim and free of bloat when it's time to put on a bikini.

2. Skip sun damage. Enhance your antiaging sun defenses from the inside with UV-protective foods like tomatoes, carrots, watermelon, apricots, and greens that contain lycopene and beta-carotene, phytochemicals that help block UV damage in the skin. Don't forget a natural mineral-based sunscreen (see Resources, page 200) and a great pair of UV-filtering sunglasses.

3. Get outdoors. Enhance your summertime beauty by taking your exercise routine outdoors, where you'll boost self-esteem and lift your spirits. You can rev up your mind and body by heading toward water; the negative ions that concentrate near waterfalls, river rapids, and waves improve your mood and energy. Make contact with the earth by walking barefoot on grass or sand, a "grounding" technique that actually balances the electrical energy of your body to reduce inflammation and increase calm.

4. Lighten up. Although summer is the season of abundance, you'll naturally crave lighter dishes. Even if raw food doesn't suit you during other seasons, give it a try during the summer. Incorporate more fresh, raw foods into your day and you'll taste the living beauty nutrition they offer.

5. Sweat better. Find a natural deodorant that allows your body to perspire (an essential form of beauty detox!), but keeps you feeling fresh. Conventional antiperspirant-deodorant formulas block natural detox and usually dose your body with toxic aluminum and paraben preservatives. See Resources, page 200, for a few of my favorite natural formulas.

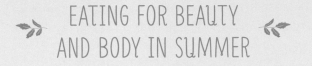

EATING FOR BEAUTY
AND BODY IN SUMMER

It's June: get yourself to a farmers' market! Seriously, if you haven't branched out from the grocery store aisles by now, it's time. The beauty food party is happening outside, and during the summer you can find Eat Pretty foods that are not only local and organic (read: higher in beauty nutrition), but priced less, if you only look around at what's growing in your area. To get even more budget-friendly, plant a garden of your own, whether it's a windowsill herb garden or a plot of summer veggies. Don't stop there—plant flowers as well, and bring cut flowers indoors to celebrate nature. Be part of the living, growing celebration of the earth this season.

Summer has signaled a shift in our routines since childhood; now channel that expectation into your grown-up intentions. Wake up with the sun on summer mornings, slice a fragrant lemon in half, and squeeze the detoxifying juice of one half into a glass of warm water to lay the groundwork for beauty all day (use room-temperature water if warm is unappealing in summer months). A green smoothie is my summer pick to feed beauty first thing in the a.m. Blend fresh greens and the juice of your remaining lemon half with your choice of beautifying fats and proteins: avocado, chia, almond butter, hemp, and spirulina are top picks. A few hours into the morning, you'll be ready for a snack, so have a little protein like a hard-boiled egg with a summer beauty food like berries, or pop some spirulina tablets (amazing for energy and a clear complexion).

At lunch and dinner, shift your Eat Pretty diet to focus on foods that prevent and repair damage in the body. Your skin, hair, and nails are healthy and happy at the start of the season, but it's important to maintain that beauty with plenty of nutrient-rich age-defense foods. Eating foods rich in carotenoids and vitamin C—foods like yellow and red bell peppers, cantaloupe, and papaya—maintains healthy collagen in your skin and blocks UV damage. At midday especially, keep hydration in mind; it's important for digestion, immunity, and detoxification. Hydrate with anti-inflammatory and naturally cooling foods like cucumbers, watermelon, zucchini, and coconut water. Water-rich foods like these can be a better source of hydration for the body than water alone. All throughout the day, drink purified water, and sip chilled herbal teas like mint and hibiscus. Limit dehydrating caffeine and alcohol, and moderate your spicy foods, which can overheat your body before they eventually cool you down.

Eating lighter is a good strategy for supporting your small intestine this season, since the digestive tract undergoes natural cleansing when it has sufficient time to rest between meals. You also don't want to create heaviness or indigestion in the body during hot weather. As you'll learn in Chapter 9, taking a probiotic supplement can support good digestion year-round.

Summer and its fire element signal a time of communication and connection; this season social opportunities abound. Instead of picking up a bag of chips or a pack of hot dogs to bring to a barbecue, make an Eat Pretty dish that you'll feel good about eating and sharing. Or host a pampering summer gathering filled with Eat Pretty foods and beautifying smoothies.

Summer is packed with natural desserts: berries, stone fruits, melons, and tropical treats. It's also a time of frosty, sugar-packed cocktails, ice cream, popsicles, and processed snacks tossed into beach bags and backpacks. For your beauty, go the naturally sweet route. If there is a single season to steer clear of Beauty Betrayer foods like processed snacks and sugary frozen desserts, it's summer. Refined sugar, alcohol, and charred foods create AGEs—stiff, wrinkle-causing proteins (see page 24). The more AGEs hanging around in your skin, the more susceptible you are to damage from UV rays.

The Eat Pretty
❧ SUMMER BEAUTY BASKET ❧

Summer fruits, veggies, and herbs are Eat Pretty foods at their best! This colorful crop brims with beautifying powers, from UV defense and collagen building to natural cooling and hydration. Dig in and get your summer glow on. For more information on the beauty nutrients in these foods, refer to the Beauty Nutrients chart (page 46) and Phytochemical Beauty Boosters chart (page 51).

APRICOTS: Beta-Carotene Booster

Apricots have a rather short season, so snatch them up when you see them fresh at your local market. Ripe apricots are full of beta-carotene (four apricots deliver about 60 percent of your recommended daily intake), making them must-eat beauty foods! Their UV-protective vitamin A nourishes beautiful hair, nails, and smooth skin, and their phytochemical zeaxanthin supports healthy eyes. Apricots are a surprising source of the beauty minerals iron and copper, as well as the mineral potassium for hydration balance. They're great digestive aids, and even have mild laxative properties. Dried apricots are a concentrated source of sugar, so choose fresh instead (they'll fill you up), or stick to just two or three unsulfured, naturally dried halves.

EAT PRETTY FOOD	BEAUTIFYING COMPOUND	BEAUTY BENEFIT
Apricots	Vitamin A	Supports smooth skin

BLUEBERRIES: Look (and Think) Like You're Twenty Again

When it comes to blues, go easy on the eyeshadow and fill up on the berries. On the surface, blueberries may not look powerful, but their deep blue skins contain a stable of antiagers that keep you looking, thinking, and seeing like a spry young thing. Specifically, anthocyanin pigments boost skin's elasticity and connective tissue (bye-bye sagging) and protect against UV damage, while catechins defend against wrinkles. Vitamins C and E top the list of the more common beauty nutrients in blueberries (they're even more powerful in concert, since C helps regenerate E in the body), and their healthy dose of potassium boosts the circulation of nutrients and oxygen. They may even help reduce fat storage in your body, thanks to their ability to decrease insulin resistance. Eat them fresh or frozen, but not dried, for the biggest benefits.

EAT PRETTY FOOD	BEAUTIFYING COMPOUND	BEAUTY BENEFIT
Blueberries	Anthocyanins	Boost skin elasticity

CANTALOUPE: A and C for the Day

Cantaloupe combines two major beauty vitamins, A and C: just 1 cup/ 170 g has more of both A and C than you'll need in a full day! A and C are powerhouse prevention against acne, wrinkles, sun damage, lackluster skin, and dry scalp. Cantaloupe also has plenty of potassium to keep your body hydrated and your beauty nutrients circulating, aided by vitamin B$_6$, which keeps sodium and potassium balanced in your body. Those B vitamins are also key for healthy, lustrous hair. Cantaloupe is one of the few foods that contain a high potency of an enzyme called superoxide dismutase that supports mitochondrial health. For optimal digestion, eat your cantaloupe by itself, or at least thirty minutes before a meal.

EAT PRETTY FOOD	BEAUTIFYING COMPOUND	BEAUTY BENEFIT
Cantaloupe	Vitamin A	Protects against UV damage

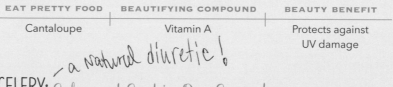

– a natural diuretic!

CELERY: Calm and Cool in One Crunch

Why does celery make you feel as slender as, well . . . a celery stick? Its healthy balance of sodium and potassium makes it a natural diuretic, with the power to cool, detox, and flush your body of excess fluid. Celery is just what you need when you're feeling a little too hot and heavy in the summer heat. And as you're cooled by celery, you're calmed, too, thanks to the phytochemical coumarin and its blood pressure–lowering properties. Celery's content of silicon supports skin elasticity and hydration, plus healthy hair growth (silicon is one ingredient in a popular over-the-counter hair-growth supplement)—a good reason for you to snatch some off a platter of crudités. As you crunch away, remember that celery also defends against inflammation and wrinkles.

EAT PRETTY FOOD	BEAUTIFYING COMPOUND	BEAUTY BENEFIT
Celery	Sodium	Maintains electrolyte balance

CHERRIES: *Inflammation Defender*

Whether you like them deep ruby red or cheerful yellow-pink, cherries are bursting with antioxidants that keep your body looking and feeling young. The pigment molecules called anthocyanins in cherries, like those in blueberries and plums, help firm skin and keep connective tissue strong and youthful, plus they protect DNA from oxidative damage. The antioxidant quercetin in cherries helps prevent UV damage; it's also an antihistamine that may reduce allergy symptoms. Cherries are powerful anti-inflammatory foods, used to alleviate arthritis and soreness after workouts, and they're important for blocking wrinkles caused by inflammation and reducing skin redness. Sweet cherries, the larger varieties we most often see in the grocery store, offer a good dose of vitamin C and potassium. And tart cherries, a more medicinal variety, provide even more C, plus a potent dose of beta-carotene. Tart cherries are one of the few foods that contain natural melatonin, which regulates sleep cycles to give you a better night of beauty rest.

EAT PRETTY FOOD	BEAUTIFYING COMPOUND	BEAUTY BENEFIT
Cherries	Anthocyanins	Strengthen skin and connective tissue

COLLARD GREENS: *Major Nutrition, Minimal Calories*

Collards are a member of the powerhouse *Brassica* genus of beauty veggies. Like their relatives Brussels sprouts and cabbage, collards are a good source of potent cancer-preventative compounds called glucosinolates, which also boost the body's production of the antiaging nutrient glutathione. Collard greens are low in calories (only about 11 calories in a big handful of chopped leaves), yet they contain plenty of beta-carotene that converts to beauty vitamin A for healthy hair, skin, nails, and eyes, and a hefty dose of collagen-building vitamin C. With their deep green color, collards are rich in chlorophyll to oxygenate your blood; vitamin K for blood vessel health; and folate, important for red blood cell production and healthy pregnancy. Eat them raw in a smoothie or salad, or lightly steam them for a beautifying side dish.

EAT PRETTY FOOD	BEAUTIFYING COMPOUND	BEAUTY BENEFIT
Collard greens	Glucosinolates	Boost antiaging glutathione

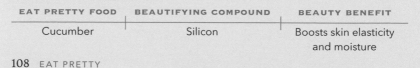

buy organic & eat them with the skins!

CUCUMBER: *Cool as Ever*

When it's hot outside, cucumbers are like a cool breeze for your body and beauty. They're rich in silicon, a beauty mineral that's essential for healthy connective tissue and skin moisture and elasticity; and they're packed with water (95 percent!) for a hydration and detoxification boost. The potassium in cucumbers keeps beauty nutrients circulating, while magnesium keeps you calm (and together, research shows, these two chemicals may lower blood pressure). Cucumbers are anti-inflammatory, kidney-cleansing foods that prevent water retention and keep your body slim. They're surprisingly good sources of vitamin K, and super-low in calories (an entire cucumber contains only 45). It's worth buying organic cucumbers so you can eat them with the skins, which are good sources of vitamin C and chlorophyll.

EAT PRETTY FOOD	BEAUTIFYING COMPOUND	BEAUTY BENEFIT
Cucumber	Silicon	Boosts skin elasticity and moisture

OKRA: Smooth Digestion Secret

The slippery gel inside an okra pod is its most memorable trait—and rightly so, since the gel, called mucilage, gives it unique detoxifying benefits. The mucilage in okra feeds healthy bacteria and lubricates the intestines, making it a digestion and elimination booster. Mucilage also helps keep blood sugar steady by preventing the rapid absorption of sugar in the digestive tract. Fewer blood sugar spikes means less inflammation and acne. While you're at it, you'll be getting a well-rounded dose of B vitamins for healthy circulation and strong hair and nails.

EAT PRETTY FOOD	BEAUTIFYING COMPOUND	BEAUTY BENEFIT
Okra	Mucilage	Feeds healthy digestive bacteria

PAPAYA: Anti-Inflammatory Sun Shield

It's no surprise that this sunny orange fruit bursts full of age-fighting vitamin C; there's about one and a half times your recommended daily intake of C in 1 cup/225 g of the tender flesh. Together with its natural dose of vitamin E, beta-carotene, and lycopene, papaya protects skin from signs of sun damage, like wrinkles and brown spots. Even more beautifying: papaya contains a digestive enzyme that reduces aging inflammation and promotes healthy digestion of proteins, as well as phytochemicals thought to protect from cancer. Papaya seeds may have hidden health benefits themselves; these edible, peppery seeds are said to cleanse the intestines.

EAT PRETTY FOOD	BEAUTIFYING COMPOUND	BEAUTY BENEFIT
Papaya	Lycopene	Defends against UV damage

PEACH: Complexion Dream

If you really want a peaches-and-cream complexion, fill up on this, vitamin C– and beta-carotene–rich fruit. You probably know by now that C is one of the most powerful free-radical fighters, and is essential for the manufacture of healthy collagen to keep your complexion smooth and youthful. The beta-carotene in peaches converts to vitamin A, the beauty vitamin that helps with regular cell repair and exfoliation. Peaches contain a small dose of vitamin E, which strengthens the cell membranes for healthy skin and scalp. Peaches also help with cooling the body, as well as circulation, digestion, and fluid retention, so they're a welcome snack in the summer heat.

EAT PRETTY FOOD	BEAUTIFYING COMPOUND	BEAUTY BENEFIT
Peach	Vitamin C	Boosts collagen production

PEPPER: C is for Collagen

Bell peppers Red/yellow/Orange have more beauty benefits than green

You can't really go wrong when choosing your favorite pepper, but keep these two bits of beauty info in mind: red, yellow, and orange bell peppers have more beauty benefits than green bell peppers, and hot peppers, like poblano, chile, and jalapeño varieties, contain much, much more of the antiaging phytochemical capsaicin found in the white membrane inside the pepper. Whether you go sweet or hot, all peppers support good circulation. But peppers with higher levels of capsaicin are especially anti-inflammatory, chemoprotective, circulation-boosting—and antiaging. Capsaicin suppresses a cell signal that starts a chain of inflammation and aging processes in the body. Sweet bell peppers only have trace amounts of capsaicin, but they're extremely high in collagen-building vitamin C. One sweet yellow pepper has about 600 percent of your daily vitamin C needs. Sweet bell peppers are also great sources of B vitamins for healthy hair and antiaging beta-carotene (especially the phytochemical lycopene) for firm, elastic skin. Rinse peppers in cold water and eat them raw to keep their delicate antioxidants intact.

EAT PRETTY FOOD	BEAUTIFYING COMPOUND	BEAUTY BENEFIT
Pepper	Capsaicin	Reduces inflammation

PINEAPPLE: Flat-Belly Favorite

This sweet tropical treat contains a powerful anti-inflammatory digestive compound that breaks down protein and boosts overall digestion. Pineapple's enzymes combine with its insoluble fiber to help you maintain a flat belly and less bloat when you eat it fresh (in moderation, since it's high in natural fruit sugar). Pineapple is rich in vitamin B_6 and copper, two nutrients for healthy hair and hair color; plus potassium, for circulating beauty nutrients around the body. Pineapple also balances water and heat in the body, making it a wonderful summer food!

EAT PRETTY FOOD	BEAUTIFYING COMPOUND	BEAUTY BENEFIT
Pineapple	Vitamin B_6/pyridoxine	Supports healthy hair color

PLUM: Antioxidant Treasure

Sweet summer treat—and potent age fighter? Plums fit the bill. They're a cooling food, perfect for hot weather, that (like prunes, a type of plum) have natural laxative effects. Plums may match or even exceed the antioxidant value of blueberries, and they offer anti-inflammatory and even antiobesity defenses. Plums contain anthocyanins, which defend against collagen breakdown, and their other phytochemicals have even been shown to inhibit breast cancer growth. Eat them at their ripest, juiciest point, when antioxidant levels are highest.

EAT PRETTY FOOD	BEAUTIFYING COMPOUND	BEAUTY BENEFIT
Plum	Anthocyanins	Protect collagen and skin firmness

RASPBERRIES: Biotin Booster

These delicate, gem-like berries contain an impressively large list of antioxidants, from collagen-protecting anthocyanin pigments to toxin-fighting ellagic acid. Raspberries also offer age-fighting, collagen-building nutrition from vitamin C and plenty of fiber for their small size. The raspberry has blood-building and liver-supporting properties that strengthen and support gorgeous skin and healthy hair, plus biotin that's important for growing hair and nails. Its high content of manganese also helps the body preserve mitochondrial health.

EAT PRETTY FOOD	BEAUTIFYING COMPOUND	BEAUTY BENEFIT
Raspberries	Vitamin B$_7$/biotin	Strengthens hair and nails

TOMATO: Sun-Defense Star

There's nothing quite like a vine-ripened summer tomato, so get your fill while they're in season! Eating tomatoes while the sun shines has another beauty benefit: the anti-cancer nutrients lycopene and beta-carotene in tomatoes defend the skin from UV damage that causes wrinkles, age spots, and lines. Eating tomatoes regularly concentrates this photoprotective benefit in skin. Cooking tomatoes increases lycopene absorption, as does a little drizzle of olive oil—the natural pairing to ripe summer tomatoes that provides vitamin E to amplify the damage-preventing actions of vitamin C. Tomatoes are also anti-inflammatory and high in potassium, to keep your electrolytes in balance for healthy circulation of beauty nutrients.

EAT PRETTY FOOD	BEAUTIFYING COMPOUND	BEAUTY BENEFIT
Tomato	Lycopene	Defends against UV damage

WATERMELON: Sweet and Slimming

Watermelon is a long, hydrating drink of water for your skin (really—92 percent of every bite is H$_2$O). The antioxidant lycopene in watermelon gives your body strong UV-defense properties that work in tandem with your sunscreen to keep you sun-damage-free all summer. For summer slimness, watermelon reduces water retention and cools and detoxifies the body. It's a surprising source of iron—important for red blood cell production, which leads to healthy hair, pretty pink nail beds, and radiant skin. It also helps the body make arginine, an amino acid that is indirectly involved in bodily healing and the production of antiaging HGH. Arginine supports cardiovascular health, ensuring healthy blood flow throughout the body.

EAT PRETTY FOOD	BEAUTIFYING COMPOUND	BEAUTY BENEFIT
Watermelon	Iron	Maintains healthy red blood cell production

ZUCCHINI: Low-Cal, High C

Not only is zucchini—and yellow squash, a zucchini variety—a seriously low-cal veggie (just 20 calories in one small zucchini), its fiber and detoxifying pectin make you feel full and block absorption of even more of its calories. But don't think the beauty benefits of zucchini are bland. Zucchini offers a dose of antiaging vitamins C and A, plus relaxing, blood pressure–lowering magnesium and potassium. You'll also find beauty nutrients like B_6 and folate for healthy hair, and riboflavin for collagen building, in every bite.

EAT PRETTY FOOD	BEAUTIFYING COMPOUND	BEAUTY BENEFIT
Zucchini	Magnesium	Calms nervous function

➤➤ SUMMER AT A GLANCE ◀◀

With these Eat Pretty foods for summer beauty, you're about to make this radiant season come alive. Eating for beauty will support you, protect you, and energize your every cell so that you can relish the abundant beauty of summer, without draining your body or compromising your skin, hair, nails, and waistline. Have fun with summer beauty foods, experiment with new recipes, and let nature inspire you.

SWEET SUMMER COOLER

You'll want to serve this refreshing and deeply hydrating drink on the hottest summer days. To save time, you can swap in pineapple juice and bottled coconut water, but you'll always get more beauty benefits from fresh, unprocessed pineapple and coconut water straight from a young coconut. As a splurge, it makes a great base for a summer cocktail.

Serves 4 to 6

8 stalks celery

½ fresh pineapple, cut into large chunks (or 8 oz/240 ml pineapple juice)

2 young coconuts (or 20 oz/ 600 ml bottled coconut water)

Using a juicer, extract the celery and pineapple juice. Pour the juice into a large pitcher. Open the young coconuts and drain the water into the pitcher. Stir to combine and chill until ready to serve.

BLUEBERRY LENTIL SALAD

This vibrant summer salad is packed with alkalinity, vitamin C, antioxidants, and DNA defenders, plus it's beautiful to behold. If assembling the salad ahead of time, leave out the watercress until just before serving.

Serves 6

1 cup/200 g dried millet, rinsed and drained

Sea salt

¾ cup/145 g dried green lentils, rinsed and drained

1 bay leaf

1 organic red bell pepper, seeded and finely chopped

1 heaping cup/170 g organic blueberries

¼ cup plus 2 tbsp/90 ml olive oil

2 tbsp raw unfiltered apple cider vinegar

2 tbsp umeboshi plum vinegar

½ tsp dried dill

¼ tsp dried oregano

Freshly ground black pepper

1 bunch watercress

Put the millet in a saucepan and add water to cover and a large pinch of salt. Bring to a boil, reduce the heat, and simmer, uncovered, for about 15 minutes, until the millet is tender but still retains a slight crunch. Remove from the heat, drain excess water, and set aside to cool.

In another saucepan, combine the lentils and 1½ cups/360 ml water. Add the bay leaf and bring to a boil. Reduce the heat and simmer for about 25 minutes, or until the lentils are tender but not mushy. Drain any excess water and set aside to cool.

In a large bowl, combine the millet and lentils, bell pepper, and blueberries. In a separate bowl, whisk together the olive oil, vinegars, dill, oregano, and season with salt and pepper. Pour over the salad and toss to coat. Chop the watercress leaves and about 2 in/5 cm of the stems. Toss into the salad just before serving.

SWISS CHARD AND TOMATO FRITTATA

This dish makes a protein-packed brunch entrée, served warm—or cold, straight from the fridge. It's one of my favorite recipes for healthy nails, especially if you use omega-3–rich pastured eggs.

Serves 6

1½ tsp coconut oil
1 leek, white and light green parts only, chopped
5 large Swiss chard leaves, stemmed and roughly chopped
1 tomato, seeded and chopped

2 garlic cloves, minced
8 eggs
1½ tsp capers, drained
Sea salt and freshly ground black pepper

Preheat the broiler.

In a 9-in/23-cm cast-iron frying pan, melt ½ tsp of the coconut oil over medium heat. Add the leek and cook until soft and golden, about 5 minutes. Add the chard, tomato, and garlic and cook until the chard wilts, about 4 minutes longer. Pour off any liquid and transfer the veggies to a plate.

Wipe the pan clean, add the remaining 1 tsp coconut oil, and melt over medium-low heat. Meanwhile, in a large bowl, beat the eggs and capers with a large pinch of salt and pepper. Starting with the cooked chard mixture, alternate layers of the veggies and the egg mixture in the warm greased pan until you have used all of both.

Cover and cook the frittata for about 5 minutes, until the edges are set. Transfer to the broiler and cook, uncovered, for about 5 minutes, or until lightly browned on top. Remove from the oven and loosen the edges with a knife. Let the frittata cool slightly before loosening further with a spatula and sliding onto a serving plate—or serve straight from the pan.

GREEN WRAPS WITH TILAPIA, PINEAPPLE, CUCUMBER, AND SUN-DRIED TOMATO PESTO

Assemble all of the ingredients beforehand so you can roll and serve these wraps as soon as the fish comes off the grill.

Serves 4 to 6

1 cup/55 g sun-dried tomatoes, rehydrated in water and drained
1 tsp red curry paste
½ cup/120 ml vegan natural mayo
Leaves of 2 fresh oregano sprigs
10 large collard leaves, stemmed
½ pineapple

1 organic cucumber
2½ lb/1.2 kg tilapia fillets, or other white fish such as trout
Sea salt and freshly ground black pepper
2½ cups/80 g sprouts such as mung beans or alfalfa

In a food processor, combine the sun-dried tomatoes, curry paste, mayo, and oregano and process until well combined. Using a sharp paring knife, shave down any thick areas of the central spines of the collard leaves, taking care not to tear them. Cut the pineapple into thin strips and the cucumber into thin rounds.

To prep the wraps, place the collard leaves, spine-side down, on a work surface. Top each leaf with about 1 tbsp of the sun-dried tomato pesto. Arrange the pineapple and cucumber slices on top, dividing them evenly.

Heat the grill to medium-high. Rinse the fish, pat dry, and season with salt and pepper. Wrap in aluminum foil, place on the grill, and cook for 8 to 10 minutes, or until the fish is opaque throughout and flakes easily (open a packet to test with the tip of a knife). Divide the fish among the wraps and top with the sprouts. Form each wrap by folding the sides of the leaf over the filling and rolling up the bundle bottom to top like a burrito. Serve warm.

CHAPTER 7

RESTORE AND RECHARGE IN AUTUMN

The days shorten, sunlight wanes, the air gets crisp, and a chill sets in. Can't you just feel the summer glow draining from your complexion? No need to fear the onset of flaky, pale skin, chipping nails, or dull, dry hair this fall, because you'll be filling up on autumn's freshest foods to deliver the nutrition your body needs to radiate beauty from the inside out. The juicy, antioxidant-rich fruits and berries of summer may be in short supply, but there's a colorful new crop of beauty foods ripe for the picking. Your skin won't lack beauty nutrition during this season of abundant harvest. With a full spectrum of autumn beauty foods to explore, you'll maintain your healthy summer radiance over the cool months ahead.

If summer's intense heat and UV exposure took a toll on your skin and hair, fall is the ideal time to repair and revive your beauty. The good news: the foods in your autumn beauty basket reduce damage, fight signs of aging, and address autumn skin concerns like dryness all at once. It's no coincidence that fall beauty foods are amazing at repairing damage and restoring the body. Did you know that apples, one of our favorite fall foods, are powerful detoxifiers that work to cool your body from the lingering heat of the summer? Or that pumpkin, a must-have fall veggie, is packed with vitamin A to boost cell turnover and nourish beautiful hair, nails, skin, bones, and teeth? Those are just two of the autumn beauty foods that you'll meet as you eat your way through this chapter of cozy, comforting—and above all, beautifying—autumn foods.

In the beauty industry, the arrival of fall coincides with fashion week, when designers present their upcoming collections, and suddenly there is a huge focus on trends. What lip color will everyone be wearing next season? Will the hair on the runway be blown straight or teased into a beehive? After a few years of having an insider's view of backstage beauty at fashion shows, I realized that, season after season, one thing is certain: you'll never have to worry about hitting or missing a beauty trend if you show up with a healthy glow. Whether or not you're a follower of the trends you see in fashion magazines, there's no question that well-nourished skin, hair, and nails and a healthy body make you a beauty inspiration worthy of any runway.

In the fall we also return to the grind of work and school, leaving the lazy days of summer behind. It's normal to feel your stress level rising as deadlines and commitments pile on, so you'll want to keep things calm and cool inside and out by increasing your intake of foods that fight the effects of stress (pay special attention to B vitamins, magnesium, and omega-3s). Chronic stress creates inflammation, the un-pretty immune response that leads to visible signs of aging like wrinkles and sagging skin, plus redness, irritation, and blemishes. An inflamed body is more susceptible to disease, weight gain, fatigue, and accelerated aging inside and outside.

Eastern traditions link the fall season to the lungs and the large intestine, two organs that take in nourishment (the former from air and the latter from food) and release what we do not need. This is an ideal time of the year to be more mindful about two particular beautifying practices: deep breathing and thorough chewing. These seemingly natural impulses are easy to let slip in the distraction and stresses of modern life, but they are key to providing ample nourishment for our bodies. The release of air and food by our lungs and large intestine mirrors our release of the beautifying foods and energy of

> ⚘ **BEAUTY EDITOR NOTE** ⚘
>
> *Deepen your hydration from the outside with organic body oils from some unexpected Eat Pretty foods—try avocado oil, sweet almond oil, or plum kernel oil and apply from scalp to cuticles.*

summer. And autumn supplies its own healing, grounding foods (you'll find so many amazing beauty foods this season!) that help us transition to a new season of beauty.

EATING FOR BEAUTY AND BODY IN AUTUMN

Getting out of bed is even harder as the days get darker, and on autumn mornings you probably don't feel like the bundle of energy you were during the sunnier months. Continue to start each day with a cup of warm lemon water to support healthy liver function and good digestion, which keeps a bright, healthy glow in your skin. At times you'll also want to warm up with tea for detoxification and hydration. Green tea has an amazing ability to stop the function of enzymes that cause skin wrinkling, and its health benefits increase when you drink it with a squeeze of lemon. (See more of my favorite teas for beauty on page 128.)

The light, cooling smoothies of summer may be enough breakfast to satisfy you early in the fall season, but you'll begin to crave warm, hearty meals to start the day as we move deeper into autumn. That gives you the perfect reason to eat more grains that are rich in fiber and beauty minerals that sustain you on chilly mornings. I find that gluten-free grains like millet, buckwheat, amaranth, and protein-packed quinoa are the most beautifying—and the most versatile. Cook them in big batches and use them for on-the-go breakfasts, lunches, and dinners throughout the week. You can even freeze cooked grains if you find yourself jet-setting out of town before they're used up!

Depending on the climate in your area, autumn days can feel like an extension of summertime—or a wake-up call that winter is on its way. It's helpful to have go-to recipes for a few lighter dishes that can be served hot or cold, depending on the temperature that day. This fall your best friend for beauty nutrition could be the Autumn Beauty

Your AUTUMN Beauty Intentions

Starting a new season with a focus on your beauty intentions for the months ahead gives you a clear course toward your beauty and health goals. Keep a copy of this list where you can refer to it all season long to turn these short-term goals into long-term beauty habits.

1. **Do damage control.** Fill up on autumn beauty foods rich in healing nutrients (sweet potatoes, red cabbage, pumpkin, and broccoli are great picks), and you'll give your body the tools it needs to repair and rejuvenate your skin after a long, hot summer. Autumn beauty foods are particularly rich in vitamin A, one of the most restorative nutrients for your skin, hair, and nails.

2. **Skip the sugar.** Refined sugar is the number one food enemy of a youthful complexion, so be choosy when faced with baked goods and sweets during the holidays. When a celebration (or sweet tooth) calls, whip up a batch of skin-friendly Pumpkin Spice Pudding (page 137), Cool Peppermint Cream Cups (page 157), or a few Oatmeal-Raisin Cookie Truffles (page 76) to share.

3. **Get grounded.** When we're stuck indoors during the autumn and winter months, it's easy for our bodies to lack a connection to the earth. Many people find that root vegetables like sweet potatoes, turnips, and beets ground their energy and provide a feeling of strength and stability during the colder seasons.

4. **Light your digestive fire.** Improving your digestion will strengthen your beauty and immunity for the months ahead. Take a daily probiotic (see page 171), snack on fermented foods (see page 170), and make my Cranberry-Orange Beauty Sip, a sweet-tart digestive tonic: Blend 1 cup/100 g of raw cranberries with 1 cup/240 ml of purified water, half a peeled and seeded orange, and a generous shake of cinnamon. When you eat a meal, chew each mouthful well—twenty to thirty times if you can—to break down food in your mouth and lessen the load on the rest of your digestive system.

5. **Let go of Beauty Betrayers.** Autumn is the season of letting go. Instead of falling into beauty-busting (and diet-busting) habits that take a toll on your appearance during the holidays and leave you feeling regretful come January 1, let go of Beauty Betrayer foods now, and be proud of your decision to nourish your beauty all year long.

Bowl (page 136), a recipe that you can throw together in minutes and customize to suit your cravings, the farmers' market foods that are freshest, or the leftovers you have in the fridge.

Fall piques your appetite for warmer, heartier dishes, and the foods in this chapter are full of grounding qualities and beauty nutrition to feed your radiant looks and warm up your body. These beautifying meals are especially comforting and sustaining, just what our bodies need during the fall; but they won't overfill you or spike your blood sugar, leaving you drowsy or low in energy. Try not to eat your dinners late at night, so your body stays free to rest and repair as thoroughly as possible without using up extra energy on nighttime digestion. During the fall and winter, a hot water bottle is one of my favorite ways to warm up, ease digestion, and boost circulation before bed.

And the sweet finale: treats are inescapable this season, as fall holidays make way for an avalanche of December festivities. While I do love desserts, I don't love the effects that an overload of refined sugar has on my skin: visible blemishes, redness, irritation, eczema, and AGEs, which will cause wrinkles in the years to come. Splurging on Eat Pretty fall sweets (try the Pumpkin Spice Pudding on page 137 for your fall flavor fix) gives you both instant and delayed gratification, as you maintain a youthful complexion in the weeks ahead. Has there ever been a better reason to try a new dessert?

> ✒ **BEAUTY EDITOR NOTE** ✒
>
> *For smooth skin, one of my favorite exfoliating masks is raw honey alone, which loosens dead skin cells, attracts moisture to skin, and reduces blemish-causing bacteria. Leave it on clean skin for 20 minutes before rinsing.*

The Eat Pretty
❧ AUTUMN BEAUTY BASKET ❧

Stock these autumn beauty foods for the next three months (and beyond, if you're lucky enough to get a bumper crop from the fall harvest in your own garden or the farmers' market) for the most grounding, beauty-boosting, nutritious foods and flavors of the season. For more information on the beauty nutrients in these foods, refer to the Beauty Nutrients chart (page 46) and the Phytochemical Beauty Boosters chart (page 51).

ACORN SQUASH: *Beauty-Mineral Gold Mine*

You need a variety of beauty minerals for the healing processes of your body to run smoothly and energetically—and acorn squash can help. This sweet squash is high in minerals, making it a powerhouse hair and nail booster. Iron in acorn squash keeps hair and nails from becoming brittle and thin, while its vitamin C helps your body use iron to its fullest. Acorn squash offers plenty of B vitamins like niacin, key for circulation and DNA repair, and thiamine and pantothenic acid, both important for healthy metabolism. Calcium and magnesium are two minerals in acorn squash that are important for healthy bones and teeth, so you can stand tall and flash a gorgeous smile.

EAT PRETTY FOOD	BEAUTIFYING COMPOUND	BEAUTY BENEFIT
Acorn squash	Iron	Strengthens hair and nails

APPLE: *All About the Skin*

You probably see the same three or four types of apples at the market—that is, until the autumn harvest arrives. Crisp fall apples are not only a treat to bite into, they're a serious fall beauty staple. They come in dozens of varieties and taste incredible eaten straight from the tree or the farmers' market. During the autumn season, apples are prized for their ability to detox and cool the body from summertime heat. Apple skins contain the antioxidant, anti-inflammatory pigment quercetin, which has become a hot skin-care ingredient for its powerful defense against free-radical and UVB damage. As you might guess, quercetin carries equally impressive benefits internally—as an anti-cancer and antiaging compound, and a natural antihistamine. Apple skins also contain a phytochemical that defends against wrinkle-causing AGEs. Apples are a great source of pectin, which fills you up, helps the body detoxify, and even lowers cholesterol. And new research is being done on the ability of apples to balance bacteria in the large intestine—certain to be a big plus for your digestion and your skin. An apple a day keeps the breakouts at bay?

EAT PRETTY FOOD	BEAUTIFYING COMPOUND	BEAUTY BENEFIT
Apple	Quercetin	Defends against free-radical damage

BROCCOLI: Secret Inflammation Buster

Broccoli—one of the veggies that most frequently get pushed to the side of the plate—should be front and center in your beautifying diet. Broccoli is an amazing source of collagen-building, wrinkle-preventing vitamin C; bone-reinforcing calcium and potassium; and vitamin K to strengthen capillaries and prevent dark circles and varicose veins. Phytochemicals called glucosinolates in broccoli regulate detoxification at a genetic level throughout the body. Research shows the glucosinolates actually increase after light steaming, so you don't always need to crunch your broccoli raw. Broccoli also contains a phytochemical called indole-3-carbinol, which reduces the risk of estrogen-sensitive cancers like breast, cervical, and ovarian. All this, plus it contains the phytochemical sulforaphane, which helps prevent stress-related inflammation in the body. Eating your broccoli has really never been more glamorous.

EAT PRETTY FOOD	BEAUTIFYING COMPOUND	BEAUTY BENEFIT
Broccoli	Sulforaphane	Prevents stress-related inflammation

BUTTERNUT SQUASH: *Healthy Hair Secret*

This sweet and oddly shaped squash is absolutely brimming with beta-carotene, which converts to vitamin A—a powerful vitamin to heal and smooth your skin, decrease UV sensitivity, and protect your scalp and eyes. If your skin looks lackluster this season, peel and cube butternut squash and roast it for an instant beauty-boosting side dish. The complex B vitamins in butternut squash are excellent for hair health, since they help your body produce red blood cells that nourish gorgeous locks. Butternut squash is also a good source of vitamin E, iron, and (surprisingly!) omega-3s, all of which are important for healthy hair follicles and a well-hydrated scalp. Roast the seeds for a dose of tryptophan, an amino acid that's a precursor to calming serotonin.

EAT PRETTY FOOD	BEAUTIFYING COMPOUND	BEAUTY BENEFIT
Butternut squash	Beta-carotene	Heals and smoothes skin

CHARD: *Nailing It with Biotin*

Want the hair and nails of a storybook princess? Strengthen both from the inside with biotin-rich chard. Biotin (vitamin B_7) helps the body use protein, which is critically important for repairing damage and keeping skin, hair, and nails strong and healthy. A biotin deficiency can actually cause hair loss, so make chard a regular green in your beauty diet. Of course, you'll get more than just biotin from chard leaves. Calorie for calorie, dark, leafy greens like chard deliver one of the most concentrated sources of beauty nutrition. Chard is full of vitamins A and C, two nutrients that are essential for cell repair and healing after a long summer of damage, as well as vitamin E for UV protection, vitamin K and calcium for healthy bones, and lutein, a critical nutrient for eye health that may also decrease wrinkles.

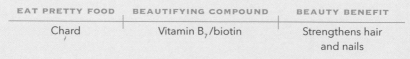

EAT PRETTY FOOD	BEAUTIFYING COMPOUND	BEAUTY BENEFIT
Chard	Vitamin B_7/biotin	Strengthens hair and nails

CRANBERRIES: Raw Antiaging Power

Raw, organic cranberries surpass sugar-filled jellied cranberry sauce in every beautifying way imaginable. Fresh cranberries are absolutely packed with antioxidants (surpassed only by blueberries), including anthocyanin pigments that protect our cells and collagen, and lower aging inflammation. Flavonoids in cranberries, like the powerful quercetin, increase the skin's tolerance to UV light and give the skin a gorgeous glow by increasing blood flow to the skin. Cranberries also keep us beautiful by promoting good digestion and healthy lymph flow and preventing urinary tract infections.

EAT PRETTY FOOD	BEAUTIFYING COMPOUND	BEAUTY BENEFIT
Cranberries	Anthocyanins	Lower wrinkle-causing inflammation

DAIKON RADISH: Crunchy Cleanser

This giant radish is odd-looking, but don't let its appearance keep you from experiencing the peppery crunch and big beauty benefits within. Daikon is a traditional Japanese vegetable that cools the body, detoxifies the liver and stomach, and decongests the lungs. It's packed with enzymes that ease the burden on your regular digestion, leading to better assimilation of nutrients and less bloating—both of which mean clearer skin and healthier beauty head to toe. Daikon is also a good source of iron, made more absorbable by its vitamin C, for healthy circulation and strong hair.

EAT PRETTY FOOD	BEAUTIFYING COMPOUND	BEAUTY BENEFIT
Daikon radish	Enzymes	Boost digestion and assimilation

ESCAROLE: For Antiaging, Bitter is Better

Here's one way to go green with your beauty routine: eat escarole, a slightly bitter, leafy green that's full of skin-smoothing vitamin A, as well as about

Build a BEAUTIFYING TEA APOTHECARY

Tea offers so much more than warmth and hydration. Steep the right teas and you'll relax, be better equipped to fight off a cold, feel more energetic, and, yes, defend against wrinkles! For the biggest beauty benefits, I always recommend tea over coffee. A few of my favorite teas for healthy vanity:

Chamomile tea protects your skin from sun damage, thanks to its high concentration of the phytochemical quercetin, and promotes restful sleep and cramp relief during your period.

Dandelion root tea is a gently diuretic brew that supports liver function and digestion, both of which are essential for gorgeous skin!

Ginger tea, or an infusion of fresh grated ginger root, chases away colds, helps you digest heavy meals, and works beauty magic as a powerful anti-inflammatory for your body and skin.

Green tea has the ability to block wrinkle formation and even reverse UV damage, thanks to its free radical-fighting catechins like EGCG. The catechins in green tea are even more powerful antioxidants than vitamins C and E, and they've demonstrated the amazing ability to restore and revive dying skin cells.

Rooibos, or red tea, is brimming with antioxidants, including quercetin, the UVB-protectant pigment that's anti-cancer, antiaging, and—bonus for allergy sufferers—a natural antihistamine.

Tulsi tea helps the body handle stress and balance hormones with its soothing, energizing powers. Some of my favorite tulsi blends combine the herb with ginger, jasmine, and rose.

White tea contains anti-inflammatory phytochemicals that prevent the breakdown of collagen and elastin in the skin, which directly contributes to signs of aging. White tea offers antiaging effects even in small amounts, so you can feel beautiful about sipping just one cup.

30 percent of your recommended daily intake of collagen-building vitamin C. Escarole is also a great source of dark circle–reducing vitamin K, iron, calcium, and folate, a powerful nutrient for healthy DNA synthesis. The powerful A, C, K combination in escarole means you're getting an antiaging boost with every bite. Escarole's cousin, radicchio, also offers cooling, toning beauty benefits after the heat of the summer.

EAT PRETTY FOOD	BEAUTIFYING COMPOUND	BEAUTY BENEFIT
Escarole	Vitamin K	Reduces dark circles

FIGS: *Fruit of Love*

If figs live up to their rumored aphrodisiac properties, it's because they contain amino acids that help boost blood flow to the skin and, well, other areas of the body. Fresh figs contain natural digestive enzymes that give your body a break, plus plenty of fiber (think of all those little seeds) that has a gentle laxative effect for easy elimination. These delicate little jewels, both fresh and dried, are rich in beauty minerals, especially manganese, calcium, potassium, and magnesium. Figs are also one of the rare fruits to contain antiaging omega fatty acids in their seeds, and they're highly alkaline fruits that keep your pH balance in check.

EAT PRETTY FOOD	BEAUTIFYING COMPOUND	BEAUTY BENEFIT
Figs	Amino acids	Boost blood flow to the skin

GRAPES: *Go Red for Antiaging*

Grapes come in many colors, but it's the deep red and purple grapes that seem to offer the most beautifying powers. Grapes are anti-inflammatory, reduce water retention, and have strong antioxidant phytochemicals that keep blood vessels healthy and beauty nutrition flowing throughout your body. Resveratrol, just one of those phytochemicals, is concentrated in the skin and seeds of grapes. In nature, resveratrol defends the grape plant against bacteria and sun damage—not too far off from the defensive role it appears to have in our bodies, as an extender of cell lifespan. Research suggests that resveratrol can slow the aging process in our cells and protect DNA by activating a particular gene that controls longevity. It may also boost energy production in our mitochondria, keeping us young and energetic. Grapes do contain lots of sugar, so enjoy a few at a time, to sweeten a fall smoothie or as a frozen treat.

EAT PRETTY FOOD	BEAUTIFYING COMPOUND	BEAUTY BENEFIT
Grapes	Resveratrol	Protects DNA and slows aging

KOHLRABI: Friendly Fiber

These hard, round, green-and-purple veggies look puzzling to some, but they're just one more *Brassica* genus member with big beauty benefits. Like their cousins Brussels sprouts and turnips, kohlrabi are endowed with glucosinolates, which aid in liver detox and break down into sulforaphane, a phytochemical that lowers inflammation, defends against DNA damage, and lessens redness and UV damage. Kohlrabi is full of anti-aging antioxidant defenders, like collagen-building vitamin C, potassium for healthy blood flow, and a wide range of B vitamins that strengthen hair and red blood cell production. It's also packed with fiber for digestive health and blood sugar stability, two must-haves for happy, glowing skin.

EAT PRETTY FOOD	BEAUTIFYING COMPOUND	BEAUTY BENEFIT
Kohlrabi	Glucosinolates	Support liver detox

LEEK: Cell Defender

Leeks are a member of the powerhouse *Allium* genus (along with garlic, onions, scallions, and chives) whose phytochemicals stimulate the production of the mega cell-protective antioxidant glutathione, the body's most critical antioxidant. Glutathione protects the mitochondria of our cells, prevents and repairs DNA damage, lessens sun damage, and boosts the body's elimination of toxins. Leeks contain the anti-cancer phyto-chemical kaempferol, and also help stop collagen-digesting processes that would otherwise cause wrinkles and signs of aging in the skin.

EAT PRETTY FOOD	BEAUTIFYING COMPOUND	BEAUTY BENEFIT
Leek	Glutathione	Powerful antioxidant defender

PUMPKIN: All-Around Beauty

Just a cup or so of antioxidant, anti-inflammatory pumpkin purée has enough beta-carotene to deliver seven times the recommended dietary allowance for vitamin A. What does this mean for your looks? You'll be boosting your beauty head to toe, as vitamin A is crucial for beautiful skin, hair, nails, bones, and teeth. Pumpkin's lutein and zeaxanthin protect eyes from aging free-radical damage, and its high fiber and natural diuretic properties detoxify and reduce water retention so you'll always fit into your skinny jeans.

EAT PRETTY FOOD	BEAUTIFYING COMPOUND	BEAUTY BENEFIT
Pumpkin	Lutein	Protects eyes from aging damage

PUMPKIN SEEDS: Your Clear Skin Companion

Pumpkin seeds are one of the best plant-based sources of zinc, an essential anti-inflammatory beauty mineral that encourages hair growth, strong nails, and clear skin. Low levels of zinc are commonly found in acne sufferers, so make pumpkin seeds a regular snack if you have breakout woes. They reduce *Propionibacterium acnes*, which, as the name implies, are bacteria that cause blemishes. Pumpkin seeds are a good source of the amino acid tryptophan that helps produce calming, relaxing serotonin in the body, so make them a go-to snack before bedtime, or when you're feeling anxious. Pumpkin seeds also contain a long list of antiaging nutrients like omega-3s, vitamins A, B, and K, and the minerals niacin, magnesium, iron, and copper.

EAT PRETTY FOOD	BEAUTIFYING COMPOUND	BEAUTY BENEFIT
Pumpkin seeds	Tryptophan	Produces calming serotonin

RED CABBAGE: Beauty Never Smelled So Sweet

The vibrant purple pigment in red cabbage leaves comes from anthocyanins, phytochemicals that are full of free radical–fighting power and have the power to neutralize enzymes that break down connective tissue. Add that to the fact that red cabbage is a fantastic source of collagen-building vitamin C (it packs almost twice the amount of C as green cabbage) and you've got a major beauty food. Red cabbage also packs in the fiber, vitamin K, vitamin B_6, and silicon, an oft-overlooked beauty mineral that may protect your hair and nails against breakage. Don't forget the anti-cancer association of red cabbage: it's one of several cruciferous vegetables that contain glucosinolates, which are natural sulfur compounds (they give cabbage its signature smell) linked to prevention of cancers like breast, colon, and prostate.

EAT PRETTY FOOD	BEAUTIFYING COMPOUND	BEAUTY BENEFIT
Red cabbage	Vitamin C	Builds collagen

SHIITAKE MUSHROOMS: It's Elastic

Shiitake mushrooms are known for their immune-boosting properties—so much so that one of the most powerful nutrients in shiitakes is approved as an active ingredient in a mushroom-based anti-cancer drug used in Japan. On the beauty side, shiitake mushrooms reduce inflammation and prevent DNA damage, and they're full of iron, B and D vitamins, and selenium, a trace mineral that protects our skin's elasticity.

Shiitake mushrooms also contain estrogen blockers that evidence has shown may lower your risk of breast cancer.

EAT PRETTY FOOD	BEAUTIFYING COMPOUND	BEAUTY BENEFIT
Shiitake mushrooms	Selenium	Maintains skin elasticity

SWEET POTATO: Eat Your ABCs

The orange tint of sweet potatoes is a dead giveaway: these tasty root vegetables are full of beta-carotene, an antioxidant pigment that converts to the powerful beauty vitamin, A. Just 1 cup/225 g of cooked sweet potato packs an amazing 769 percent of your daily needs for vitamin A, along with fantastic doses of vitamins C and B, especially B_6. Vitamin A keeps skin smooth and cell division running smoothly, regenerates collagen, and maintains your beauty head to toe, from hair and teeth to bones and nails. Vitamin C is another important vitamin for collagen production, while B_6 is especially important for healthy hair and beauty sleep. This complex carb will keep you feeling satisfied without a glycemic spike that could contribute to blemishes. Yams, which are often confused for sweet potatoes, offer fewer beauty nutrients, so make sweet potatoes your top choice!

EAT PRETTY FOOD	BEAUTIFYING COMPOUND	BEAUTY BENEFIT
Sweet potato	Vitamin A	Repairs and smoothes skin

❧ AUTUMN AT A GLANCE ❦

Nature may be turning inward to prepare for the months ahead, but your new autumn beauty tools keep your beauty energetic and radiant. The beauty foods you'll eat this season will warm your kitchen; feed your skin, hair, and nails; and deeply ground and sustain your body during a busy season.

WARM FALL SALAD WITH CRANBERRY-GINGER VINAIGRETTE

This salad packs in some of fall's most beautifying foods: sweet potatoes, apples, cranberries, and ginger. It's an antiaging boost in a bowl that you can serve to a crowd, or keep all to yourself.

Serves 4 as a main course

1 large sweet potato, scrubbed but not peeled
1 large apple, scrubbed but not peeled
2 medium carrots, peeled
1 head kale, stemmed and chopped

VINAIGRETTE:
One 2-in/5-cm piece fresh ginger
1 cup/100 g raw cranberries
½ cup plus 2 tbsp/150 ml olive oil
2 tbsp apple cider vinegar
2 tbsp balsamic vinegar
Sea salt and freshly ground black pepper

Bring about 6 in/15 cm of water to boil in a large pot. Meanwhile, chop the sweet potato and apple into ½-in/12-mm dice. Peel the carrots into 2-in/5-cm ribbons with a vegetable peeler. Set aside.

Using a steamer basket, submerge the sweet potato chunks in the boiling water until tender-crisp, about 2 minutes. Remove and set aside to drain. Using the same basket, plunge half of the kale into boiling water for 30 seconds. Remove and, using tongs, squeeze out any excess water; toss the steamed kale with the remaining raw kale in a large salad bowl. Add the sweet potatoes, apples, and carrots and toss to mix. Set aside.

To make the vinaigrette: Coarsely chop the ginger. In a food processor, combine the ginger, cranberries, olive oil, and vinegars, season with salt and pepper, and process until smooth.

Pour the vinaigrette over the salad and toss to coat. Serve warm.

RED CABBAGE SLAW WITH
SWEET AVOCADO-LIME DRESSING

The sweet, tart crunch of this cabbage slaw is addictive, and with its high water content (a cup or so of shredded red cabbage is only about 20 calories), you can go ahead and help yourself to another serving. Given its major beauty benefits—like a significant dose of vitamin C—it's a dish to feel gorgeous about serving all year long.

Serves 4 to 6

5 cups/325 g thinly sliced red
  cabbage
2 cups/200 g shredded
  daikon radish
1 large handful of finely chopped
  fresh parsley
1 ripe avocado, pitted and peeled

3 tbsp fresh lime juice
5 tbsp/75 ml water
¼ tsp ground maca
4 drops liquid stevia
Sea salt
¼ cup/40 g dried unsweetened
  cranberries

In a large bowl, toss together the red cabbage, radish, and parsley. Set aside.

In a food processor or blender, combine the avocado, lime juice, and water and process until smooth. Add the maca and stevia, season with salt, and blend to incorporate. Add the dressing to the slaw and toss to mix and coat well. Top with the cranberries and serve.

AUTUMN BEAUTY BOWL

Farro is not a gluten-free grain, but it is low in gluten and there-fore more easily digestible to those with intolerances. Those with serious gluten allergies should substitute a fully gluten-free grain like quinoa or millet.

Serves 2

1 cup/185 g warm cooked farro
2 tbsp fresh lemon juice
3 tsp coconut oil
1 medium shallot, minced
1 cup/100 g thinly sliced
  daikon radish
3 tsp minced fresh sage leaves,
  plus a few whole leaves for
  garnish

4 oz/115 g shiitake mushrooms,
  stems removed, tops brushed
  clean and chopped
4 oz/115 g cremini mushrooms,
  brushed clean and chopped
5 tsp wheat-free tamari
One 8-ounce/225-g package
  tempeh

Toss the cooked farro with the fresh lemon juice and set aside. In a large frying pan over medium heat, melt 1 tsp of the coconut oil. Add the shallot and cook until softened, about 2 minutes. Add the radish and 2 tsp of the sage and cook, stirring, for 2 minutes longer. Add the mushrooms, sprinkle with 2 tsp of the tamari and cook, stirring occasionally, until the mushrooms are tender, about 10 minutes.

    Meanwhile, in a small frying pan over low heat, melt remaining 2 tsp coconut oil with the remaining 3 tsp tamari. Raise the heat to high. Add the remaining 1 tsp sage, crumble in the tempeh, and cook until heated through and slightly browned, about 5 minutes.

    To serve, toss together the farro and veggies, top with tempeh, and garnish with the sage leaves.

PUMPKIN SPICE PUDDING

The beauty nutrition in this pumpkin pudding makes it a guilt-free indulgence. For added beauty benefits, top individual servings with bee pollen or chopped walnuts.

Serves 4

1½ cups/350 g cooked pumpkin
   or butternut squash purée
1 frozen banana (peel before
   freezing)
1 cup/240 ml unsweetened
   almond milk

¼ cup/40 g flaxseed
1 tbsp pure maple syrup
2½ tsp Eat Pretty Pumpkin Pie
   Spice (recipe follows)
1 tsp ground cinnamon
1 tsp vanilla extract

Using a high-powered blender, combine the pumpkin, banana, almond milk, flaxseed, maple syrup, pumpkin pie spice, cinnamon, and vanilla and blend on high until smooth, 60 to 90 seconds. Serve immediately, or chill for 30 minutes or longer for a thicker texture.

❧

Eat Pretty Pumpkin Pie Spice

Shake this beautifying spice blend into smoothies, on cereal, into baked desserts and pudding, or anywhere else you want an anti-aging, fall-flavor kick. Makes 3½ tbsp.

2 tbsp ground cinnamon
2 tsp ground ginger
1 tsp ground cloves

1 tsp ground allspice
1 tsp ground nutmeg

Put the cinnamon, ginger, cloves, allspice, and nutmeg in a small bowl and mix well. Transfer to an airtight container and store up to 1 year.

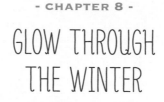

- CHAPTER 8 -

GLOW THROUGH
THE WINTER

The month of December holds some of the biggest holidays of the year, but the winter solstice, on December 21, isn't one of them. It arrives quietly, almost unnoticed—a sweeping contrast to the energetic party that takes place six months earlier at the summer solstice. Winter has a beauty all its own, and sometimes it takes a little searching to find.

In a word, winter beauty is "parched." It's a quest for hydration from your scalp to the tips of your fingernails, in an effort to escape dry, chapped skin, flare-ups of eczema and rashes, and lines and wrinkles that appear more prominent in cold temperatures. Our bodies slow down for the winter season and, suddenly, we need to work a lot harder for the basic moisture, circulation, and cell turnover that happen effortlessly in warmer months. In addition to all the healthy and hydrating foods you'll be eating this season, keep a natural hand cream and face mist at your desk or in your purse to keep your hands soft and your complexion dewy. Winter beauty also means immunity, since it's next to impossible to look and feel your best if you're fighting a cold or the flu. Good news: Eat Pretty winter beauty foods keep your immune defenses strong, and help prevent the dreaded red nose, eye bags, chapped lips, and achy exhaustion of illness.

In addition to the cold, dry temperatures, winter brings a nutrition roller coaster. The season starts with a burst of excess, followed by a few anxious weeks of dieting, repenting, and regretting what we failed to accomplish in the past year. How are any of us supposed to feel beautiful while caught up in that unhealthy pattern?

It's not easy to change deeply ingrained habits with hasty resolutions, but if we use our healthy vanity to stay mindful of our beauty and body, we can break out of the cycle. Let's enter this season with the intention to follow an Eat Pretty routine and make at least one beautifying choice daily, rather than make resolutions, which research says about 22 percent of us ditch within a week. By sticking to our daily rituals, we aren't thrown off track by the highs and lows of the season.

When you live the Eat Pretty lifestyle in winter, you pass by the Beauty Betrayer foods that cause inflammation and weight gain. Eliminating Beauty Betrayers helps strengthen your kidneys and adrenal glands—the organs of winter, according to Eastern tradition. The kidneys filter our blood, and our adrenals produce vital hormones for our bodies. They are two important organs of moisture, warmth, and energy, which we desperately need during the harsh winter. Supporting these organs now helps build energy for the beautiful renewal you'll experience in the spring, so adequate rest and warming beauty nutrition are powerful winter tools. It can be difficult to embrace the darkness of winter, but, without it, the spring would not appear so profoundly beautiful. Ahead, you'll find my plan for building and restoring your beauty this winter.

> ❧ BEAUTY EDITOR NOTE ❦
>
> *Don't throw away the refined sugar in your cabinet; use it to make a circulation-boosting body scrub. Mix equal parts sugar and oil (try olive or sweet almond) with a drop or two of your favorite essential oil and massage from the neck down while in the shower.*

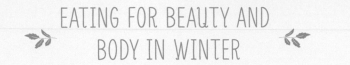

EATING FOR BEAUTY AND BODY IN WINTER

It's cold outside! Not to mention a bit gray. But you've still got a beautiful glow, because you're eating warming, sustaining beauty foods that feed your radiance and good moods from the inside.

At this time of year we could all take a lesson from nature, which stores away its beautifying energy. So many of us suffer from adrenal burnout, a result of stress, poor diet, and lack of sleep—which in turn causes fatigue, sugar cravings, headaches, anxiety, tension, and even difficulty sleeping, and takes a massive toll on our beauty and health. It's so important not to miss the ideal restorative moments that winter presents to support our adrenals with nourishing foods and rest. I'm not suggesting that you hibernate (cabin fever isn't pretty either), but getting adequate sleep, placing reasonable limits on partying and traveling, and eating whole foods and skipping refined sugar are at the core of an adrenal-supporting Eat Pretty diet.

Brighten the dark morning with a burst of vitamin C in your daily warm lemon water, and follow that with a warm, savory breakfast, like Comforting Kitchari (page 154), scrambled eggs, or probiotic-rich miso soup with greens. Cooked foods lessen the digestive burden so your body achieves an energy boost and better assimilation of raw materials to repair and maintain your beauty and health. Good digestion, as you will learn in Chapter 9, can actually prevent some of the eczema, acne, and rashes that you might otherwise struggle with during the winter.

Ideal wintertime meals for lunch or dinner are soups, stews, grain and veggie dishes, and wild salmon, sardines, or other fish rich in protein and omega-3 fats. As skin tends toward redness and sensitivity in the winter, base your meals on anti-inflammatory beauty foods. Drinking warm water or tea throughout the day encourages natural detox, increases

Your WINTER Beauty Intentions

Starting a new season with a focus on your beauty intentions for the months ahead gives you a clear course toward your beauty and health goals. Keep a copy of this list where you can refer to it all season long to turn these short-term goals into long-term beauty habits.

1. Circulate. Make sure you regularly break a sweat during the winter, to bring oxygen and nutrition to your skin, boost immunity, lower stress, detox your body, and lift your mood. In addition to a gorgeous glow, sweating stimulates the natural release of oil that moisturizes and softens our skin and scalp. You'll see a healthier complexion and glossier hair all winter long.

2. Get a shot of immunity. I don't just mean a flu shot! To naturally support your immune system, boost your vitamin C intake (with winter beauty foods like Brussels sprouts and oranges), as well as your zinc (oysters are a potent source) and vitamin D (mushrooms and sardines, or a supplement). Since refined sugar suppresses your immune system, skip it (including sugary OJ when you are feeling under the weather).

3. Take a long winter's nap. Winter is the season of deep rest, and sleep is essential for weight control, adrenal health, and overall beauty. Go to bed earlier and sleep a little longer this season. If you are having difficulty sleeping, read ahead and implement the Eat Pretty beauty sleep essentials in Chapter 9.

4. Heat things up. Warm, cooked food requires much less energy to digest than the same amount of raw food. Eat plenty of cooked foods throughout the winter, and season your foods with warming spices like cinnamon, cayenne, or ginger to encourage easy, complete digestion.

5. Make friends with fats. Even a heavy, vitamin-infused night cream isn't enough to replace a diet that hydrates your skin from within. Healthy fats (walnuts, avocados, wild salmon—you know the list by now!) shore up your skin's moisture defenses from the inside and support balanced hormones, blood sugar stability, and absorption of essential vitamins. Skipping good fats can actually make you feel colder, hungrier, and more cloudy-headed and can mess with your menstrual cycle.

your circulation, and ensures that you eliminate regularly, so you won't wind up battling bloat. Whenever possible, make your midday meal the most substantial, so you won't feel sleepy and lethargic on winter nights.

And when it comes time to party, your body will be so well nourished that you'll make better choices. With balanced blood sugar, you'll reduce your cravings for the processed sweets that age you so quickly. Since lots of holiday foods hold a sentimental significance, you might still want to pick a few foods to splurge with, and keep the rest in line with Eat Pretty. After all, a holiday party is meant to be a time to celebrate and treat your body, not test its limits or burden it with excess. The holidays are an emotional time of year, for better or worse, as you see family and friends and reflect on the past and the new year ahead. Overall, try to celebrate with foods that make you look and feel your best during the event and in the days afterward. Remember, a little weight gain is normal in the winter, so don't let it get you down or throw you off track. Be kind to your body and beauty, and build love and quality into your meals—you deserve it.

The Eat Pretty
⇉ WINTER BEAUTY BASKET ⇇

Fill your kitchen with these winter beauty foods (there's nothing bleak about them) while it's cold outside, and you'll always have the most beautifying, warming, nutrient-dense foods of the season at hand. For more information on the beauty nutrients in these foods, refer to the Beauty Nutrients chart (page 46) and the Phytochemical Beauty Boosters chart (page 51).

AVOCADO: *Mitochondrial Defender*
Avocado face masks may be all the rage, but eating avocado is far tastier—and more beautifying. If you're lucky enough to have a creamy,

ripe avocado in front of you, get your beauty boost from the inside out! Avocado is one of the healthiest sources of fats in nature, and you need those fats to stay beautiful, so add it to smoothies, salads, sandwiches, and dips whenever you can. Eat avocado in moderation (half an avocado per day is a good limit), but do not get caught up in calorie counting. Avocado burns easily for energy and fires up the natural detox processes of the liver, which helps skin stay clear. Avocados are rich in vitamin E, a powerful antioxidant vitamin that keeps skin cells strong and hydrated, and B vitamins like niacin, which assists in detox and DNA repair and reduces redness and inflammation in skin. There are about 2 g of protein in half an avocado.

EAT PRETTY FOOD	BEAUTIFYING COMPOUND	BEAUTY BENEFIT
Avocado	Vitamin E	Keeps skin cells strong and hydrated

BANANA: Digestive Darling

Bananas are known for their potassium content, which keeps beautifying nutrition and oxygen circulating, and their ability to provide fast energy, which makes them a great snack for athletes. But they enhance beauty as well as sports performance! Bananas contain an amino acid that boosts healthy hair and nail growth and protects the body from aging free radicals. They also contain silicon, an essential element for strong hair, nails, and collagen. They're easily digested and soothing to the lining of the stomach, and they feed good bacteria in your gut. Bananas also contain complex carbs that increase mood-enhancing serotonin production in the body. Since they're naturally sweet and low glycemic, bananas work very well as a sweetener in skin-friendly desserts. The riper the banana, the more antioxidants!

EAT PRETTY FOOD	BEAUTIFYING COMPOUND	BEAUTY BENEFIT
Banana	Potassium	Maintains electrolyte balance

BEETS: Double the Detox

Betalains, the phytochemicals in beets, increase the body's production of glutathione, the beautifying nutrient that detoxifies, stimulates liver cell function, and protects our mitochondria. Beets give the lymphatic system a natural boost in the winter and contain lots of detox-friendly pectin and fiber. They contain collagen-building vitamin C, iron, beta-carotene, and vitamin K to defend against bruising and support healthy bones. Beets also contain lycopene, a plant chemical that helps maintain youthful skin elasticity and defends against sun damage. Save the greens from your beets and steam them as a side dish or toss them into green smoothies as you would kale or lettuce. They're a great source of vitamins A, C, and protein that you won't want to waste.

EAT PRETTY FOOD	BEAUTIFYING COMPOUND	BEAUTY BENEFIT
Beets	Betalains	Increase glutathione production

BRUSSELS SPROUTS: DNA Defender

Like broccoli and cauliflower, Brussels sprouts are a member of the *Brassica* genus of naturally detoxifying beauty veggies. Brussels sprouts top the charts for cancer-fighting glucosinolates, many of which break down into sulforaphane, a phytochemical that lowers inflammation, protects cells from DNA damage, revs up the body's production of antiaging glutathione, and reduces redness and damage caused by UV exposure. Brussels sprouts also contain indole-3-carbinol, a phytochemical that eliminates excess estrogens, keeping hormones in balance. To release these beneficial compounds, chop or chew your Brussels sprouts well! One serving (a generous cup, trimmed and halved) of Brussels sprouts has about 160 percent of your daily vitamin C, enough to keep collagen production humming along, and about 270 percent of your vitamin K needs, to nourish healthy blood vessels and bones and regulate levels of aging inflammation.

EAT PRETTY FOOD	BEAUTIFYING COMPOUND	BEAUTY BENEFIT
Brussels sprouts	Indole-3-carbinol	Detoxes excess estrogens

CACAO: A Treat for Your Complexion

This beauty superfood has a higher concentration of antioxidants than any other food we now know of, thanks to its powerful phytochemicals like epicatechin that block the formation of wrinkles. The catechins in cacao throw a one-two antiaging punch: they turn off age-promoting cell mechanisms while activating protective cell mechanisms. Chocolate with a high cacao percentage (look for at least 70 percent) helps protect the skin from UV damage, while cacao in general boosts skin hydration and reduces skin redness by increasing nutrients, blood, and oxygen supplied to the skin. Cacao is a feel-good food that raises levels of neurotransmitters like serotonin and endorphins in the brain. It's also one of the highest dietary sources of magnesium, which calms the nervous system and regulates heart rate. Cacao contains plenty of sulfur, a beauty mineral that promotes strong hair, nails and skin. To absorb the most antioxidants from your chocolate, choose dark and dairy-free versions.

EAT PRETTY FOOD	BEAUTIFYING COMPOUND	BEAUTY BENEFIT
Cacao	Catechins	Block wrinkle formation

CARROT: A All the Way

By now you know that vitamin A is one of the most essential beauty vitamins. What should you snack on when your complexion needs a vitamin A boost? Try carrots, one of the best veggie sources of beta-carotene, which the body converts to vitamin A. Vitamin A keeps skin, hair, nails, and eyes beautiful by promoting natural cell division, regenerating collagen, regulating oil production, and slowing the natural deterioration of eyesight as we age. Carotenoids like those in carrots also appear to lower women's risk of developing breast cancer, most likely because vitamin A regulates the growth and development of cells. Carrots are also a great source of biotin, a nutrient that's important for healthy hair growth and blood sugar regulation.

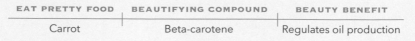

EAT PRETTY FOOD	BEAUTIFYING COMPOUND	BEAUTY BENEFIT
Carrot	Beta-carotene	Regulates oil production

CAULIFLOWER: *A Head of Antiaging*

The average cauliflower may not be vibrantly beautiful (try green and purple varieties for a bit more color), but its milky white hue reminds us of one of its primary benefits: bone-building. While cauliflower does contain some calcium, it's the vitamin K in its florets that really boosts bone health, especially if you're also getting plenty of vitamin D in your diet. Cauliflower is a great source of sulforaphane, a powerful phytochemical that turns on the production of antiaging, detoxifying glutathione in the body, and protects against disease-causing chronic inflammation. Throw in cauliflower's anti-cancer properties and its essential amino acids and you've got longevity in every bite.

EAT PRETTY FOOD	BEAUTIFYING COMPOUND	BEAUTY BENEFIT
Cauliflower	Sulforaphane	Boosts glutathione production

FENNEL: *Skin (and Stomach) Soother*

Fennel's crisp, licorice-like burst is a welcome addition to an otherwise heavy, sustaining winter meal. But the real reason to eat it all winter long goes beyond taste, to phytochemicals. Flavonoids in fennel prevent inflammation and aging by halting a series of damage-causing signals between cells. Kaempferol, another phytochemical in fennel, has been shown to prevent the formation of cancer cells. Fennel also contains the phytochemical quercetin, a UVB damage defender. And, in the interest of a flat belly and happy digestion, fennel boosts bile secretion to keep your digestion strong while remedying gas, indigestion, and bloating.

EAT PRETTY FOOD	BEAUTIFYING COMPOUND	BEAUTY BENEFIT
Fennel	Flavonoids	Prevent inflammation and aging damage

GINGER: *Keeping Cool Has Never Been Spicier*

Who would guess that one major benefit of this spicy, circulation-boosting root is that it *cools* inflammation in the body? Ginger is a powerful anti-inflammatory that reduces skin redness, fires up digestion, and soothes aches even better than your usual pain-relievers. Ginger and its phytochemical gingerol also have the potential to suppress the activation of aging cell mechanisms, keeping your skin looking its most youthful. Use fresh ginger root year-round, and don't forget its role as an antiviral, immune-boosting spice that remedies chest and nasal congestion when you're feeling under the weather. Say goodbye to red noses—and red skin.

EAT PRETTY FOOD	BEAUTIFYING COMPOUND	BEAUTY BENEFIT
Ginger	Gingerol	Suppresses aging in cells

GRAPEFRUIT: Sweet Detox

You expect grapefruit to be a great source of collagen-building vitamin C, but did you know it also contains a glutathione-producing phytochemical to support healthy beauty? Pink and red grapefruits are full of lycopene to protect skin from UV damage, which is important for antiaging even in the winter. And flavonoids in grapefruit offer anti-inflammatory benefits and improve blood vessel function, encouraging healthy blood flow to your skin, scalp, and nails. Grapefruit is a powerfully cleansing food that helps with liver detoxification and is thought to boost metabolism and aid in weight loss.

EAT PRETTY FOOD	BEAUTIFYING COMPOUND	BEAUTY BENEFIT
Grapefruit	Lycopene	Protects skin from UV damage

KALE: Beauty Bundle

It's no secret that kale is good for you (it's one of the most nutrient-dense foods on earth!), but would you believe that eating it regularly could do more for your skin than your expensive night cream? Just 1 cup/55 g kale delivers over 200 percent of your daily vitamin A (a powerful skin smoother) and 130 percent of your daily vitamin C (a major collagen builder). There's no question that A and C are two of the most important antiaging vitamins in your diet. And that cup of kale has a staggering 684 percent of your vitamin K needs, important for healthy blood vessels. Vitamins A, C, and K in kale team up to maintain moisturizing oils in your sebaceous glands. Kale doesn't skimp on beauty minerals either, from calcium (calcium from kale is more easily absorbed than calcium from milk) to potassium and iron. Kale supports detoxification in the liver, important for clear skin, and contains the phytochemicals lutein and zeaxanthin, shown to protect the eyes from aging. Last but not least, kale is cancer-preventative and buffers inflammation caused by stress. To keep kale's beauty benefits intact, lightly steam the leaves, but don't overcook!

EAT PRETTY FOOD	BEAUTIFYING COMPOUND	BEAUTY BENEFIT
Kale	Vitamin A	Boosts cell turnover

KIWI: Belly Flattener

Next time you see this fuzzy brown fruit in your grocery store, grab one or two as antiaging insurance. Kiwi's extremely high content of vitamin C (the highest in the fruit world) gives you a day's worth of C in just one fruit, for less than 50 calories. Vitamin C is one of the core beauty vitamins, for its role in collagen formation, free radical defense, wrinkle prevention, and even skin rejuvenation. Kiwi also contains an anti-inflammatory enzyme compound that helps reduce belly fat and may even improve allergies. Kiwi protects DNA from free-radical damage, and even stores some skin-friendly essential fatty acids in its seeds. For the most antioxidants, be sure to eat your kiwi when it's fully ripe.

> ☞ BEAUTY EDITOR NOTE ☜
>
> The enzymes in kiwi, pineapple, and papaya are powerful yet gentle skin exfoliants, so adding a few drops of their juice to a raw honey mask creates a natural skin-smoother.

EAT PRETTY FOOD	BEAUTIFYING COMPOUND	BEAUTY BENEFIT
Kiwi	Vitamin C	Boosts collagen production

ONION: *Winter Warm-Up*

Onions are warming foods that boost circulation and fight disease with their antiviral, detoxifying properties. They're also incredibly strong anti-inflammatory veggies that slow aging and prevent acne and cell damage. Onions belong to the *Allium* genus (think leeks, garlic, ramps, scallions), a group of antiaging foods that you absolutely must stock in your beauty food kitchen. Allicin, one of the phytochemicals in onions, starts a chain of events that stops the action of other collagen-digesting, pro-wrinkling enzymes in the body. Yellow and red onions in particular have very high levels of the phytochemical quercetin that protects skin from UVB damage and lowers cancer risk—and cooking does not affect quercetin levels. Onions are also a great source of vitamin B_6 for healthy hair and nails.

EAT PRETTY FOOD	BEAUTIFYING COMPOUND	BEAUTY BENEFIT
Onion	Allicin	Defends against wrinkles

ORANGE: *Skin-Friendly Sweet*

Forget candy canes and chocolate hearts—oranges (and tangerines, and clementines) are nature's winter beauty candy. But skip the orange juice, a concentrated source of sugar that leaves out many of the beauty benefits of the whole fruit. Oranges are mega-high in one of our must-have antiaging vitamins, C, and they contain detoxifying pectin fiber that can help shed pounds. Don't feel the need to pick away every spot of the white membrane, called the pith, when you peel an orange; it's rich in antioxidant flavonoids that boost immunity and help your body absorb plant-based iron. Oranges also contain phytochemicals that decrease the skin's sensitivity to light and boost circulation, bringing nourishment and a radiant glow to your complexion. And if you find yourself feeling brighter and more energetic after peeling an orange, it's natural aromatherapy: the fragrant essential oils are known to lift your mood, calm nerves, and ease depression.

EAT PRETTY FOOD	BEAUTIFYING COMPOUND	BEAUTY BENEFIT
Orange	Flavonoids	Boost immunity

POMEGRANATE: Beauty Food of Love

It's not hard to see physical beauty in this ruby-colored fruit, which has historically been a symbol of wealth, fertility, and abundance. But its beauty isn't just skin deep; it's the nutrition found *inside* that gives the pomegranate its remarkable antiaging, antiwrinkle powers. The phytochemical ellagic acid in pomegranates prevents aging inflammation in the body and stops a damaging chain of events in our cells that breaks down collagen and sets the stage for wrinkles to form. Pomegranates also protect our natural levels of nitric oxide, a chemical that keeps our circulatory systems young by boosting blood flow to organs and cells. The deep red juice of a pomegranate contains more antioxidants than blueberries, green tea, or red wine, and is said to be a powerful cleanser of lymph and blood, for the clear, radiant skin that we want all winter long. Pomegranate is also being studied for anti-cancer properties, especially in relation to prostate cancer, so share it with the guys in your life.

EAT PRETTY FOOD	BEAUTIFYING COMPOUND	BEAUTY BENEFIT
Pomegranate	Ellagic acid	Defends against collagen breakdown

POTATO: Beauty Mineral Magic

When you eat potatoes, make sure their benefits aren't completely buried under Beauty Betrayers. This spud gets a bad rap if you prepare it in one of its un-pretty forms, like French fries, potato chips, hash browns, and loaded-with-cheese-and-bacon baked potatoes. To get the most beauty from your potatoes, eat them organic with their fiber-packed skins, and skip the frying, which usually adds trans fats. From one medium potato, you'll get about a third of your antiaging vitamin C, potassium, and vitamin B_6 for the day, plus additional beauty minerals like iron, magnesium, manganese, copper, and phosphorus. Lucky for your lustrous locks that the nutrients B_6, iron, manganese, and copper are especially important for strong, vibrant hair.

EAT PRETTY FOOD	BEAUTIFYING COMPOUND	BEAUTY BENEFIT
Potato	Vitamin B_6/pyridoxine	Supports healthy hair and hair color

TURNIP: 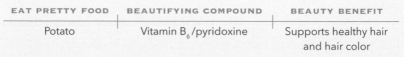 Inflammation Fighter

The turnip is a member of the *Brassica* genus, along with beauty veggies like broccoli and Brussels sprouts. Its biggest beauty benefits come from sulforaphane, an amazing antiaging compound that can stop stress-related inflammation from reaching chronic status in the body. Glucosinolates in turnips and their greens get converted to sulforaphane when they break down, so chew them well. A recent study found that the sulforaphane in turnips and other *Brassica* vegetables could fight leukemia, and the phytochemical is already known to reduce redness and damage caused by UV exposure. Turnips are full of fiber that helps with satiation and detox and they're naturally high in vitamin C. Their greens also pack plenty of C, as well as vitamin A and calcium, so be sure to eat those, too!

EAT PRETTY FOOD	BEAUTIFYING COMPOUND	BEAUTY BENEFIT
Turnip	Sulforaphane	Reduces redness and UV damage

WALNUTS: 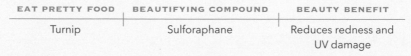 Supple Skin Snack

Raw walnuts are full of beautifying fat, protein, and minerals that guard our skin and hair against harsh, dry winter weather. Just 1 oz/30 g of walnuts has more antioxidants than the average person (but not an Eat Pretty eater, of course) consumes in a day. They're one of the few plant sources of skin-strengthening omega-3 fatty acids, converted from alpha-linolenic acid.

Walnuts are also full of beauty minerals, including zinc for healthy skin and scalp and calming magnesium, plus they're a source of hard-to-find antioxidant, anti-inflammatory phytochemicals and a uniquely beautifying type of vitamin E. They help boost our circulation of beauty nutrients by producing nitric oxide for healthy blood flow to the skin and providing iron for oxygenated blood. And, while you might have heard the myth that nuts pack on the pounds, eating walnuts in moderation (a serving is about fourteen halves) is not linked to gaining weight. All you'll be gaining is a concentrated source of major beauty nutrients.

EAT PRETTY FOOD	BEAUTIFYING COMPOUND	BEAUTY BENEFIT
Walnuts	Alpha-linolenic acid	Provides skin-strengthening omega-3s

WINTER AT A GLANCE

There is so much to celebrate this season, and you now have the tools to revel in happy occasions in ways that heal, restore, and honor your body and beauty, rather than stress and compromise them with Beauty Betrayers. You'll create new holiday traditions that help you look and feel your best, which is truly something gorgeous to celebrate!

COMFORTING KITCHARI

Kitchari is a traditional detox dish. It's warming, nourishing, and easy to digest—a perfect winter breakfast or lunch. I created this version filled with anti-inflammatory, antiaging spices and beauty foods that give it natural sweetness.

Serves 6

1 cup/220 g split yellow mung beans
1 cup/215 g long-grain brown rice
1 tbsp organic butter
2 tsp peeled and grated fresh ginger
1 tsp ground turmeric
¼ tsp ground cinnamon
⅛ tsp ground fennel
⅛ tsp ground black pepper
½ tsp sea salt

1 bay leaf
1 large sweet potato, scrubbed and cut into ½-in/12-mm cubes
2 large stalks celery, sliced ⅛ in/3 mm thick (preferably with a mandoline)
2 cups/480 ml vegetable broth
3 cups/720 ml water
Unsweetened shredded coconut for garnish

Rinse and drain the beans and rice until the water runs clear. In a medium saucepan, melt the butter over medium heat. Add the ginger, turmeric, cinnamon, fennel, pepper, and salt and stir to form a paste. Add the beans and rice and stir until coated. Add the bay leaf, sweet potato, and celery. When the mixture gets hot, add the broth and water. Bring to a boil, then reduce the heat to low. Simmer for 25 to 30 minutes, or until the rice and beans are tender. Serve topped with the shredded coconut.

ROASTED CITRUS SALAD

Take advantage of winter's beautifying citrus bounty with this refreshing salad. It's a light, crisp dish that will lift your mood with its bright flavors.

Serves 4 as a side dish

8 leaves romaine or oakleaf
  lettuce
1 bulb fennel
2 blood oranges
½ grapefruit
Melted coconut oil for drizzling

VINAIGRETTE:
3 tbsp fresh citrus juice (orange,
  lemon, or grapefruit), plus ½ tsp
  citrus zest

2 tbsp olive oil
½ tsp peeled and grated fresh
  ginger
Sea salt and freshly ground black
  pepper

Arils (seeds) of 1 pomegranate
  for garnish

Preheat the broiler.

Chop the lettuce. Using a mandoline or a sharp chef's knife, slice the fennel very thinly. Cut the oranges and grapefruit into ½-in/12-mm rounds, remove the peel, and break the slices into bite-sized chunks, leaving a few whole rounds for presentation. Line a baking sheet with aluminum foil and spread the citrus pieces in a single layer. Drizzle with coconut oil and toss to coat. Broil for 5 to 7 minutes, or until just browned.

Meanwhile, make the vinaigrette: In a small jar, combine the citrus juice and zest, olive oil, and ginger; season with salt and pepper; and shake to combine.

Combine the roasted fennel and citrus and the vinaigrette in a large salad bowl and toss to mix. Sprinkle with the pomegranate arils and serve.

WINTER VEGGIES WITH LEMON-HONEY GLAZE

The classic lemon-honey pairing gives these naturally sweet root vegetables a hint of tartness, and the addition of fennel supports digestion. Tossing the veggies in a little coconut oil helps your body absorb plenty of fat-soluble beta-carotene and convert it to vitamin A for serious skin repair.

Serves 4 to 6

5 medium carrots, peeled
2 medium parsnips, peeled
1 medium butternut squash, peeled and seeded
1 lb/455 g Brussels sprouts
2 tbsp coconut oil, melted
1 tbsp fennel seeds
½ tsp ground fennel
¼ tsp ground star anise
¼ tsp ground cardamom
¼ tsp sea salt
⅛ tsp ground cloves
2 tbsp very thinly sliced organic lemon peel
¼ cup/60 ml lemon juice
1 tsp organic lemon zest
2 tsp raw honey

Preheat the oven to 400°F/200°C. Cut the carrots, parsnips, and squash into 1-in/2.5-cm cubes, and cut the Brussels sprouts in half lengthwise. Put the veggies in a large bowl.

Combine the melted coconut oil, fennel seeds, ground fennel, star anise, cardamom, salt, and cloves in a small bowl and stir to mix. Pour over the veggies. Add the lemon peel and toss to coat evenly. Spread the dressed veggies evenly on a rimmed baking sheet lined with aluminum foil and roast until tender, about 30 minutes. Remove from the oven and let cool for 5 minutes. Meanwhile, stir together the lemon juice, lemon zest, and honey in a small bowl. Drizzle over the veggies and serve warm.

COOL PEPPERMINT CREAM CUPS

I love the beauty benefits of these minty cream cups: a boost in metabolism, antiaging capacity, and mood.

Makes 12 cream cups, serves 6 to 8

CHOCOLATE BASE:
¼ cup/55 g coconut oil, melted
⅓ cup/20 g raw cacao powder
2 tbsp pure maple syrup
¼ tsp peppermint extract
4 drops liquid stevia
Sea salt

CASHEW CREAM:
¾ cup/110 g raw cashews, soaked in water for 4 hours, drained and rinsed
⅓ cup/85 g coconut oil, melted
2 tbsp pure maple syrup
½ tsp peppermint extract
3 tbsp unsweetened almond milk
Sea salt

To make the chocolate base: In a medium bowl, blend the melted coconut oil and cacao powder until smooth. Add the maple syrup, peppermint extract, stevia, and a pinch of salt and stir to incorporate. Set twelve silicone baking cups on a tray and spoon 1 tsp of the melted chocolate mixture into each cup. Reserve the remaining chocolate at room temperature. Place the cups in the freezer for 5 minutes while you prepare the cashew cream.

To make the filling: In a high-powered blender, combine the cashews, coconut oil, maple syrup, peppermint extract, almond milk, and a pinch of salt and blend until whipped and creamy, about 90 seconds.

Scrape down the sides and blend again to eliminate any lumps. Spoon 1 tbsp of the cashew cream atop each of the frozen chocolate rounds and smooth the tops. Drizzle the remaining chocolate over the cups and freeze for at least 1 hour. To serve, unmold from the silicone cups and let thaw for 5 to 10 minutes. If the cups soften too quickly, return to the freezer to reset before serving.

PART 3

THE ESSENTIAL
BEAUTY PLAYERS

*I*f you've reached this point in your Eat Pretty journey, you've likely read, understood, and even begun to put into practice the first two parts of this book. The power to feed your beauty and health from within is securely in your hands. Now that you have a delicious foundation for looking and feeling your best, I want to share other powerful ways for you to build beauty in your daily life. In the final part of this book, I'll take your Eat Pretty makeover a step further by giving you the tools to reinforce all of the beautifying choices you make at mealtimes. This means tuning up the other major beauty players that influence the way you look and feel from the inside out: digestion, hormone health, sleep, emotional well-being, and physical activity. Supporting these important areas of your life will deepen the beauty you're so carefully nourishing with every bite and strengthen beauty in the way you feel—nourishing an even more beautiful you.

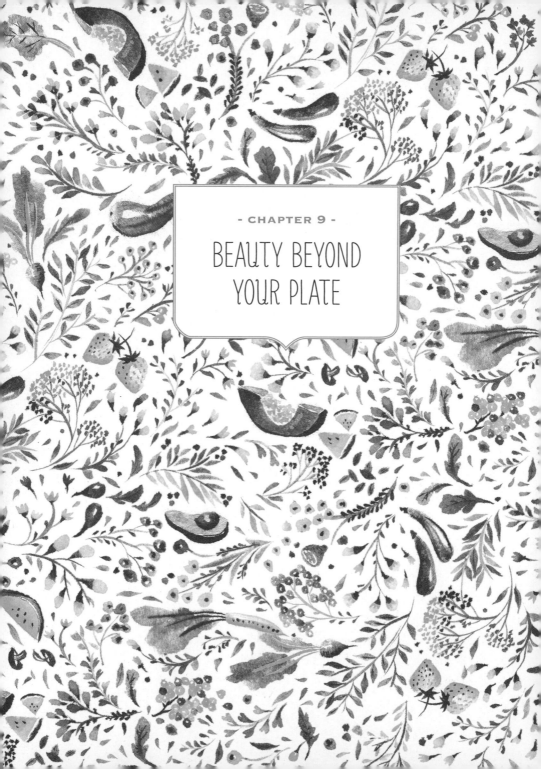

- CHAPTER 9 -

BEAUTY BEYOND
YOUR PLATE

The abundant beauty foods that fill your plate today and through the changing seasons are the firm foundation of your radiant life. They provide the energy and the raw materials to build your most beautiful body, one molecule at a time, even as they meet your seasonal beauty needs for nutrition, defense, repair, and detox. But there's more to your beauty than what you chop, cook, and chew. Beyond the foods you eat at mealtime, your thoughts and habits have the power to transform your appearance, deeply and enduringly. Your digestion determines how well you absorb beauty nutrients from your food, and influences both your immunity and your moods. Your hormone balance impacts everything from the clarity of your skin to your fertility, your energy, and the way you'll age. Your nightly hours of rest and repair can keep you slim, focused, and gorgeous, instead of triggering weight gain and cravings. And your emotional well-being and physical activity have the power to supercharge your happiness and glow. Each of these beauty players deepens your physical radiance while boosting your overall health for years to come. They're too important to overlook, but the average discussions of beauty and self-care ignore their essential roles in your beauty routine. I want you to understand these beauty players fully, as they reinforce your new Eat Pretty lifestyle, allowing your thoughts and actions to support your beauty with each bite you take.

When you combine a seasonal beauty diet with the beauty players you'll meet in the pages ahead, you'll not only gain a more complete understanding of your beauty and body, you'll see and feel a whole new level of gorgeous.

DIGESTION

Good digestion is the key that unlocks all the incredible benefits of Eat Pretty foods. Lose that key and you're barred from looking and feeling your absolute best! With the digestive tools I've outlined in the pages ahead, you'll speed up the beautiful transformation that's happening inside and out.

Eat Pretty for Optimal Digestion

If your eyes are windows to your soul, then your skin is a window to your digestive tract. When something's up down below, you notice visible clues in your complexion: dullness; breakouts (especially around your chin and on your forehead); dry, itchy patches; redness; dark under-eye circles; or some combination of the above. Your skin is irritable, and nothing you put in your mouth or on your skin seems to appease it.

Moving further inside, there are more uncomfortable hints that something's amiss, like bloating, gas, aches, cramps, rumbles and odd noises, constipation or loose stools. You know—the digestive nuisances that you hope will just disappear. Frequent colds, low moods, anxiety, or unending cravings are even more clues that you're dealing with some digestive roadblocks. Digestive troubles will take over your beauty if you let them—but you're about to find out how you can help prevent or reverse them. Get ready to get gorgeous on the outside by tuning up your inner workings.

As long as you chew and swallow your beauty foods, you can call it a day, right? Not so fast. Your digestive system breaks down and assimilates food, synthesizes vitamins and neurotransmitters, and initiates detox and elimination. Without happy digestion, your beauty nutrition isn't likely to reach your skin, hair, nails, brain, eyes, and all the other places that rely on it for beauty and vitality. What's more, the toxins that should be eliminated during digestion start to overstay their welcome when your digestion fails. I know that filling your plate with Eat Pretty foods at every meal can feel like a big task on its own. But if you could do just *one more thing*, supporting your digestive health would be it. Your reward? An even more significant shift in the way you look and feel!

There's no magic involved in the digestive process, but it retains an air of mystery simply because it happens behind closed doors. Even experts who study digestive function haven't fully unlocked all the secrets to digestive health. Here's what you, the Eat Pretty eater, need to remember: your lifestyle, your emotions, your food choices, and your eating habits influence the state of your gut and its ability to perform beauty-supporting functions. When we talk about your "gut," we mean your entire digestive system, including your stomach, intestines, and the organs that support digestion, like the liver. They all factor into the healthy beauty equation.

Every one of you healthy beauties would benefit from a gut tune-up to get the most from your Eat Pretty diet. Just a little extra attention to your digestive system can lead to a visible boost in the way you look and feel. Better digestion means more than just youthful, calm, radiant skin. It deepens your beauty with stronger immunity so you'll get sick less; better absorption of nutrients that give your hair and nails strength and resilience; healthy internal bacteria that help you stay slim and protect you from obesity and disease risk; and increased production of mood-boosting brain chemicals.

Digestion isn't the prettiest of processes, and its role in beauty gets overlooked while we rush around getting facials and shopping for a cream that promises to transform our skin from the outside in. But it's a core component of healthy beauty and antiaging. The foundation of your beauty starts *inside*, specifically in your digestive tract, where those beauty nutrients begin their journey to your skin, hair, and nails.

Maybe you've never really considered your digestion. It seems to work all right, although an upset stomach, a bout of bloating and gas, or a few days of constipation pop up now and then. No big beauty blunder, right? Not so, since digestive troubles like food allergies, acid reflux, overgrowth of harmful bacteria, and Irritable Bowel Syndrome (IBS) can cause inflammation, acne, reactive skin, and deficiencies in major beauty nutrients. Without proper digestion, even Eat Pretty foods create a toxic internal sludge that compromises our overall health, beauty, and youth. This makes digestive health one of the most important barometers of your health and beauty. It impacts the way you look and feel today, and the way your body will perform tomorrow.

Expect to hear plenty of buzz about "gut health" in the years ahead, since exploration of the human microbiome (that's the catch-all term for all the microorganisms that live in and on your body right now) is exploding. A recent study of genetic material taken from bacteria in 242 people identified more than 5 million different bacterial genes. That's pretty impressive, since we humans have only 22,000 ourselves. Our gut bacteria (we have *trillions*) outnumber our cells ten to one. That's just a small clue to their immense impact on our beauty and health. The more we understand our microbiome, the better we can treat it, and the better we'll look and feel.

The Gut-Brain-Skin Link

Stress is the single biggest obstacle to maintaining healthy digestion. To understand just how mental and emotional stresses translate to physical issues, let's look at the close interrelationship between the gut, the brain, and the skin.

Stress steadily breaks down our digestive health, and that dysfunction builds up a toxic burden that affects the beauty of our skin, as well as our physical well-being. Stressing out, whether over a deadline, a hectic commute, or a health concern, causes irritation of the intestinal walls, which results in intestinal inflammation. Inflammation compromises the function of the villi, the tiny protrusions on your intestinal walls that assimilate nutrients and start the nutrient transport process, and it clogs up the lymph drainage system that's located on the outside of your gut walls. Lymph is a detoxifying, waste-removing fluid that circulates throughout the body, and the lymph system in our gut is essential for our day-to-day detox. When it runs afoul, the lymph in the rest of our body (including the lymph that's located just under our skin) becomes inflamed, too. Soon enough, you'll see skin issues like irritation and breakouts that have nothing to do with your cleanser or moisturizer. One recent study of the gut-brain-skin axis concluded that the influence of stress and digestive health on inflammation, oxidative stress, blood-sugar control, the lipid content of tissues, and mood has important implications in acne. Isn't it time we linked digestion with radiant skin outside of the research lab as well? When our digestion isn't running smoothly, whether from compromised elimination or inflamed lymph, our liver and skin shoulder too large a share of the waste removal burden. The result is a lackluster complexion, skin sensitivity, and an onslaught of the blemishes you're working so hard to prevent.

It's particularly frustrating to me that so many acne treatment regimens involve the long-term use of antibiotics. Antibiotics and other prescription and over-the-counter drugs compromise the population of friendly flora in your intestines, and those healthy flora are exactly what we should be protecting for clear skin and a healthy body and mind! Indeed, a recent study found an association between tetracycline-class antibiotics used to treat acne and inflammatory bowel disease, particularly Crohn's disease. But this is rarely discussed. There's emerging evidence that an imbalance in your gut flora alone can cause skin issues. One study found that an overgrowth of unwanted bacteria in the small intestine was strongly linked to rosacea. Correcting the bad bacterial overgrowth resulted in a marked improvement in rosacea symptoms. Another study showed that undergoing treatment to eradicate the gut bacteria *Helicobacter pylori* resulted in an improvement or elimination of flare-ups in participants with persistent hives.

At the same time, poor digestive health takes a toll on our mental wellness. A compromised digestive system fails to produce adequate neurotransmitters like mood-boosting serotonin. Did you know that

95 percent of this chemical, which influences mood, memory, and sleep, gets produced in the gut? Low levels of neurotransmitters in the body lead to a higher risk of depression, anxiety, strong cravings, foggy thinking, and fatigue. Your gut heavily influences your mood and brain chemicals. It also controls about 80 percent of your immune system, so digestive troubles could mean increased susceptibility to illness at a time when you're already feeling down and out.

It's obvious that our gut bacteria strongly influence the beauty in the way we look and feel. In the future we can hope to see alternative therapies that use beneficial bacteria to fight infection, and keep our friendly flora healthy instead of wiping them out with antibiotics. But why wait? Read on for my favorite beautifying ways to boost your gut health today.

❧ Show some LIVER LOVE ❧

A healthy liver is one secret to gorgeous skin. For a radiant complexion, you want your liver functioning efficiently, producing bile and cleansing every last toxin from your blood. But your liver isn't able to focus on its beautifying duties if it's working overtime to pick up the slack from a compromised digestive system. Your liver gets congested when it has a to-do list full of extra detox duties because you're not digesting well, or you're eating too many Beauty Betrayer foods. A congested liver can't cleanse your blood as well as it should, which shows up in skin issues like eczema, breakouts, irritation, and a dull complexion. So give your liver a break by cutting Beauty Betrayers, and rev up efficient liver detox with warm lemon water, dandelion root or peppermint tea, and liver-loving beauty foods like artichokes.

What Goes In

Even at moments when stress feels beyond control, you can support good digestion by avoiding Beauty Betrayers—the foods that harm your beauty and health. Cooked, bleached oils and trans fats found in processed foods are a source of indigestible grease that burdens our liver. When those fats can't be efficiently filtered, they get dumped back into our bloodstream and compromise our skin health and beauty. Sugar, too, is a downer for digestive health. Refined sugar provides a feast for the harmful bacteria that can overpopulate your gut and wreak havoc on all of your beautifying digestive duties. Food allergies (think wheat, dairy, and the like) and prescription drugs also cause their own digestive troubles.

If your digestive tract is compromised by harmful foods, habits, and allergies, your body isn't assimilating and synthesizing nutrients efficiently, and your beauty is *starving*. The nutrition from our food eventually becomes muscles, blood, skin cells, bone, nerves—all the building blocks that keep our body and beauty strong and radiant. Lack of bile flow from our liver (it's stressed out—see box on facing page to see why) throws a major wrench in healthy assimilation, leading to impaired fat metabolism and lower levels of stomach acid. What happens when you're not metabolizing healthy fats and you're low on stomach acid used to break down proteins? Your skin and its lipid layer look dry and aged, and you miss out on some of the essential building blocks of your skin, hair, and nails. Gluten and casein, proteins found in wheat and dairy respectively, get broken down in the stomach, so a lack or imbalance of bile and stomach acid accounts for some of the digestive difficulty we experience from those foods. Removing them is a quick fix for our digestive health (and a boost for our beauty), but it won't solve the problem at hand. To promote healthy bile flow, try eating bile-stimulating foods like greens, radishes, and beets, and boosting your digestive fire with ginger and lemon.

If you're not digesting well, you're probably not eliminating waste efficiently either. Even if you're not constipated (which means fewer than three bowel movements a week), you could use a tune-up if you don't eliminate regularly. Your body only has so many organs that filter and eliminate: your kidneys, liver, lungs, colon, and skin. When your digestive system isn't working well, these organs pick up the slack and can become overburdened with toxins. An internal backup is just one more cause of outside beauty issues, especially dull, dry, blemished skin. Support healthy waste elimination through your digestive tract by staying well-hydrated and eating lots of plant fiber—green smoothies help you out in both departments! Just one more way to use your newfound beauty nutrition knowledge to support the healthy inner workings of your body, and your gorgeous outside.

Building Digestive Beauty

Ready to turn your gut into an efficient beauty-boosting machine? Here are my favorite ways to make digestive distress a thing of the past. Your skin will thank you.

Set the Mood

Your eating environment sets the mood for your body to receive all that gorgeous beauty food. For many of us, figuring out the best environment for our meals is the most difficult part of optimal digestion. Prep for happy digestion by drinking a glass of water to hydrate your digestive tract about 15 minutes before you plan to eat. Without this hydration, your intestinal villi won't function optimally when it's time to absorb the nutrients from your food. Hydrating before meals is also a commonsense way to avoid gulping down liquids while you eat, which dilutes the digestive juices needed to thoroughly break down your food. When eating out, sip water while perusing the menu, and you'll be well hydrated when your appetizer or entrée arrives.

As you sip that cool water, take a moment to check in with your emotions. Are you feeling especially sad, anxious, or rushed? As you assemble ingredients to prepare a meal, or scan a menu to place an order,

water before eating

your mental state matters. If you're still stressed about the pile of work on your desk, worried about your sick relative, or watching the clock to make sure you get back to the office in time for your next meeting, your body isn't completely focused on eating. Not only is it more difficult for you to make Eat Pretty choices, your body will not be adequately prepared to receive a stomach-load of food.

If you've ever had a stressful conversation over dinner, you know that stress plus food equals indigestion, and an instant stomachache. Stress shuts down deep breaths and blood flow to your digestive system, grinding the digestive process to a halt. All the more reason to eat away from your computer, or even the television, so you can focus on the beauty of your food, the powerful flavor in every bite, and the way your body responds to the foods on your plate. How can you recognize that you're full if you're scooping food with one hand while checking e-mail with the other? Set the intention to be focused, positive, and calm while you eat—and while you cook. Many cultures believe that your energy and emotions transfer to your food as you cook. It may sound a little far out, but this could also explain why a home-cooked meal, made with love, makes us feel so good.

Creating a pampering environment along with your meals is an important part of your Eat Pretty diet. That also means making peace with negative feelings about food and weight. Eat Pretty foods build your most beautiful, vital body; make an effort to receive them with joy.

A little extra focus and intention at mealtime also helps you with one of the hardest tasks around good digestion: chewing. You just can't get away with a one-two-swallow. Digestion begins in your mouth, and chewing each bite twenty to thirty times is what we *should* practice every day to absorb more nutrients. In addition to physically breaking down your food, you stimulate the release of unique enzymes in your mouth that begin the digestive process. This is why it's also helpful to "chew" your green juices and smoothies—make a chewing motion before you swallow a gulp of smoothie to get those digestive juices flowing. Any extra effort you can put in now lessens your digestive duties later, so pay it forward.

Assemble Your Secret Weapons

In addition to cutting down on sugar, allergens, and processed foods that help unwanted bacteria set up shop in your gut, stock up on foods that encourage the growth of healthy flora and smooth out hiccups in your day to day digestion. There aren't just one or two kinds of bacteria in your gut—you have a diverse ecosystem living down there. To keep your flora lush and healthy, get more of the following foods and supplements in your diet. You'll soon be wondering why you ever put up with all of those digestive rumblings:

Fermented Foods: Miso, kimchi, and sauerkraut represent distant parts of the world on our plates, but they share one important digestive booster: natural probiotics. These foods, along with brined pickles, kefir, kombucha, and tempeh, are fermented, meaning they have begun to break down in the presence of natural yeast or bacteria. The process of fermentation makes foods more easily digestible, and endows them with *trillions* of beneficial bacteria. Eating them is delicious—and helpful to your gut! When you first introduce fermented foods into your diet, start slow and give your body time to adjust, then work up to two or three small servings each day.

Herbs and Spices: Fill your kitchen cabinet with antiaging flavor enhancers that are prized as digestive aids. Ginger is the runaway favorite, for its ability to quell nausea, boost saliva flow, speed digestion, and reduce inflammation. Fennel helps relieve gas. Licorice is a natural antacid, while coriander, in concert with mint and lemon balm, has been shown to help alleviate IBS symptoms like cramps, bloating, and abdominal pain. Bitter plants like anti-inflammatory turmeric, dandelion, and gentian (found in cocktail bitters) stimulate the flow of digestive juices. And peppermint eases gas, nausea, and indigestion; try sipping it in an after-dinner tea.

Probiotics: Probiotics are supplements filled with beneficial bacteria that help your body perform its digestive duties. Probiotics are formulated to survive the early digestive process and release friendly bacteria in your intestines. Common forms are capsules, liquids and powders. When you need extra help cultivating a healthy ecosystem in your digestive tract, you can call in reinforcements with a probiotic supplement that contains billions of beneficial bacteria. At the moment, the jury's out on which type of probiotic bacteria is the most effective, so look for a mix of bacterial strains, especially *Lactobacillus* and *Bifidobacterium*. One particular strain of probiotic yeast, called *Saccharomyces boulardii*, has been linked to a reduction in acne in a scientific study. Take note, probiotics only support your good bacteria as long as you take them, so it's important to combine this tool with other digestion-boosting foods to build long-term digestive health. Look for a probiotic formula with a probiotic fiber like inulin or fructoogliosaccharides that feeds good bacteria and encourages them to colonize.

Raw Fruits and Veggies: Raw foods aren't just incredible sources of beauty nutrition; they also contain living enzymes that help your body break down and assimilate their nutrient content. Those enzymes get destroyed during cooking, so it's helpful to eat a portion of your plant foods in raw form every day. Some foods, like asparagus and leeks, have the added benefit of plant fiber that directly feeds the good bacteria in your digestive tract—yes, even bacteria need nourishment. Raw plant foods are also important because they scrub your intestinal villi with fiber and keep elimination regular, so keep eating those beautifying veggies.

Food Combining: Unlock the Beauty Combination

For optimal digestion, it's not just the foods you put in your stomach that matter, but the way you pair them—a practice called food combining. The guidelines of food combining, as you may have heard, are based on the time it takes to digest certain foods, as well as the particular enzymes needed for their digestion. There are a few different approaches to food combining, and not all of them make practical sense for our busy lives. Strict food combining means you might actually pass up fantastic beauty nutrition in order to "properly" combine. So don't sweat the rules too hard. But don't totally ignore the concept; food combining can really lessen your body's digestive burden. If you follow the three general steps below, especially at times when your digestion needs a little care, you reduce the digestive load carried by your body and free up extra energy for beauty.

1. Decide if you're having a protein-based meal or starch-based meal. If you're having quinoa, you're starching it up, and if eggs are your pick, you're doing protein. Keeping the two food categories separate helps you digest more cleanly and more easily.

2. Now, add abundant vegetables. The more the better! However, save the starchy veggies (sweet potatoes, squash, peas, potatoes) to eat with your starchy meal, not your protein meal. All the rest of the non-starchy veggies out there can be mixed and matched at will with protein-based meals and starch-based meals. You're catching on, right?

Bananas, etc

3. Fruit stands alone. Eat fruit 30 minutes before a meal, or at least two hours afterward. Fruit digests quickly, so if it hangs out in your stomach with a bunch of slow-digesting foods like protein and complex carbs, it ferments, causing (un-pretty) bloating and indigestion. One exception: foods that combine fat *and* protein, like nuts or cheese, pair happily with fruit.

eggs w/sausage pair with bananas!

Read up on optimal food combining and you'll find plenty of other rules and exceptions. This approach to eating could frustrate you, or it could offer you a creative new perspective on mealtime. Your plate isn't a quadrant to be filled with protein, fats, starch, and produce at every meal. Remember that food combining frees up energy for deeper radiance and health, even if it doesn't feel immediately necessary for your digestive system. Try it and see how you glow.

❧ AWAY FROM THE TABLE ☙

Supporting your digestion means more than just making Eat Pretty choices at mealtime. Next time you push away from the dining table, keep in mind that your breath, movement, and stress levels strongly influence your digestion as well. Both exercise and deep breathing bring blood flow to your gut, where all the action takes place, while keeping the stress hormone cortisol from mucking up the digestive process.

The Beauty of Healthy Digestion

With your digestion in good working order, you can take comfort in knowing that the beautifying nutrients in your foods are doing their jobs to transform your looks from the inside out. Of course, you can also take comfort in less bloating and indigestion, and a slimmer waistline. The boost in your beauty, body, and mood will happen faster and more dramatically with support for your digestion than they ever could with an Eat Pretty diet alone. Congratulations on making another powerfully beautifying change!

❧ HORMONES ☙

Hormones are a silent, and often confusing, factor in the state of our beauty. But we don't have to feel so out of control and in the dark about our hormone health. In the pages ahead, I'll show you how to support balanced hormones with your Eat Pretty diet and a series of pampering, beautifying lifestyle choices.

Eat Pretty for Healthy Hormones

Hormones don't take a starring role in the average beauty conversation (frankly, I think we're all hoping they'll just go away), but they're a powerful influencer of acne, weight, and aging—three areas of beauty that trouble us the most! And that's not to speak of other hormonal issues (like PMS, mood swings, painful or irregular periods, and disrupted sleep patterns) that keep us from feeling our best. Maybe you can't quite kick hormonal acne (an estimated 44 percent of us) or you just wish that you didn't feel so wiped out by stress (hmm . . . 99 percent of us?). Whatever your beef with hormones, it's time to settle the score, and build up our beauty by taking back our hormonal health.

While keeping up with the frenzied pace of a fashion and beauty magazine, I could go days (all right, weeks) without thinking about my hormones. And suddenly they'd make me stop and pay attention: I'd sink into a moody funk, burst into tears at the mention of a sad news report, and come completely unraveled under pressure of a deadline. What I didn't fully understand was that my hormones were also written all over my skin, hair, and body. I should have been paying more attention to my diet—and choosing foods and habits that encouraged my hormones to regain healthy balance. Beauties, don't make the same mistake! In your Eat Pretty lifestyle, hormone health is a top priority.

When our hormones are out of control, we don't feel our best, and we certainly don't look so hot, either. If you glance in the mirror and see breakouts, especially along your jawline and on your chin; dry and thinning skin; shedding hair; and weight fluctuations, you're looking at the top beauty-related signs of a hormonal imbalance. If you've ever noticed that a new crop of blemishes appears right before your period, when androgen hormone levels naturally rise, or that on certain days you retain enough water that your jeans won't button, then you know all too well that hormones can take a big slice of blame for beauty woes (and fashion woes, too, come to think of it). But they're not just wreaking havoc on our looks to spite us. Here's the lowdown on hormones: when you treat them well, they return the favor, especially where beauty is concerned. When kept in check, those same crazy hormones that are responsible for puffiness and hormonal acne also get at least some of the credit for elastic skin; thick, lustrous hair; strong bones; and a radiant, youthful complexion. Yes, at the right levels, hormones can actually be antiaging.

The obvious question is, how do we get hormones back on our side, and under control? How do we harness them for beauty, rather than blemishes? Ignoring them won't do. Neither will stressing out, which drives our hormones further out of balance! Time to take a deep breath, and get informed. You're about to find out why pampering yourself, Eat Pretty–style, could be your smartest prescription for hormone health.

One of my clients was led to believe that her hormones were simply a lot in life that she had to accept—completely beyond her control. How many of us fall prey to that myth? Fortunately (and sometimes unfortunately), our diets, environments, and lifestyle choices exert major influence on hormone health. Your hormones undergo natural fluctuations, but none of these shifts require you to suffer through acne flare-ups, thinning hair, or skin sensitivities. Your mission: to pamper yourself with a diet and lifestyle that restores hormone balance, using the Eat Pretty strategies outlined in this section.

Let's turn the focus inward for a few moments. Throughout this section, you'll see how greatly stress (including anger and anxiety) and Beauty Betrayers sabotage your hormone health.

Hormones and Acne

Your skin is prone to clogged pores and blemishes, and you just don't know what to do about it. Your skin-care regimen might be making matters worse, but it's probably not deserving of all of the blame. Consider whether or not there's an underlying disruptive factor working from the inside: hormones that we call androgens. Both poor diet and stress lead to an increase in androgens, hormones that happen to send sebum (oil) production into overdrive.

In addition to extra sebum, androgen hormones trigger a series of reactions that also lead to both compromised skin cell exfoliation (read: sticky, clogged pores) and inflammation, causing the red, sore blemishes we call pimples. While sebum is essential, even beneficial, for supple, youthful skin, *over*production can lead to enlarged pores, and cause a pileup of skin cells not only on the surface of your skin but within your pores. That's a recipe for uneven skin tone and the blemishes you're desperately trying to avoid! Our androgen levels increase when the body is under stress (which can also cause the skin to become more reactive, sensitive, and susceptible to outside bacteria and irritants) and when insulin is released in response to rising blood glucose, more commonly called blood sugar. A spike in blood sugar also releases the hormone that science calls IGF-1, and high IGF-1 corresponds to high sebum production and large pores.

The foods that elicit the greatest blood sugar spike are, of course, Beauty Betrayers: simple, processed carbs like breads, pasta, pretzels, sweets, alcohol—remember, they're all sugar in different forms. To keep your insulin levels in check, which is also incredibly important for preventing two growing health issues—insulin resistance and diabetes—fill your plate with foods that cause only a moderate spike in blood sugar (these are Eat Pretty foods at their best), so the amount of insulin released will be moderate as well. When too many sugar-heavy foods find their way to your lips, the insulin release is in turn much, much greater to manage the sugar rush. All of this insulin circulating in the body has negative effects on our levels of inflammation, (and, incidentally, our energy levels, as our blood sugar plummets again soon after the initial spike). Behold, your secret formula for avoiding the three o'clock energy slump, and the blemishes that come along with it: blood sugar balance!

Another major hormonal acne trigger is estrogen dominance. When the liver doesn't break down estrogen optimally, the skin can react and become inflamed. (But don't stress; supporting your liver with an Eat Pretty diet, as you learned on page 166, can help.) Adding fuel to the fire are the many skin-care products with estrogenic compounds like parabens and phthalates that have the potential to add to our already sky-high estrogen levels. In this instance, they're the opposite of beautifying.

Hormones and Weight

Wouldn't it be nice to be able to cinch your belt a little tighter? It feels so unfair that fat seems to settle around our middle, the area we most want to keep flat. What you might not know is that it's not simply overeating, but hormones released by stress and elevated blood sugar, that triggers your body to hold on to excess belly fat. When the stress hormone cortisol (designed to signal for an energy boost during your body's fight-or-flight response) stays elevated for an extended period of time (often because you're chronically stressed), it tells the body to stop burning fat, take in more food (a.k.a. stress eating), and slow metabolism. When we answer those cravings with simple carbs and sugars, up go our insulin levels, along with the storage of excess energy as fat. To add fuel to the fire, insulin suspends your fat burning ability, making it difficult to shed pounds.

Instead of feeding cravings with sugar, reach for Eat Pretty protein from plants and fish, healthy fats, and fiber-rich carbs to keep your blood sugar steady. The good news is that getting off the blood sugar roller coaster releases you from the tight hold of cravings, and as you lower your stress levels, weight may be easier to shed. Extra fat on your body releases pro-inflammatory compounds that up inflammation levels in the body and add to your aging stress burden. And keeping weight in check has the added benefit of helping to balance hormones, since stored fat acts as an endocrine organ and produces additional hormones in the body.

Hormones and Aging

As if clear skin and a slimmer waistline weren't enough incentive to balance your hormones, here's the biggest one yet: stress hormones age you prematurely. Even if other hormones stay balanced in the body, the aging processes speed up when cortisol levels remain elevated for an extended period of time. Younger bodies bounce back from the effects of cortisol within hours. But in adults, cortisol is apt to linger—making us look and feel older than we are. Stress also causes the body to produce inflammatory chemicals that lead to wrinkles, sagging, thinning skin, and fine lines, and leave you more susceptible to disease and allergic skin reactions when they hang around in the body. You'll learn more about the effects of stress on aging in the pages ahead. And of course, stressing out boosts cravings for those simple carbs (many of them Beauty Betrayer foods) that also spark an aging inflammatory response in the body—a vicious cycle. Time to halt this avalanche of aging before it begins.

Beauty in Balance

Perhaps even more meaningful than trying to understand every hormonal dip and spike is learning what we can do to restore and maintain our natural hormonal balance. Whatever your individual hormone issue may be, the Eat Pretty treatment is similar: fill your diet with beautifying seasonal foods and adopt the healthy lifestyle habits outlined in this section. They benefit every one of us, and make it easier for our beauty to flourish. Here's your hormone-healthy plan:

Eat—and Drink

There's no one food that's a magic bullet for hormone balance. But living the Eat Pretty lifestyle and eating a diet rich in beautifying foods is absolutely the place to start. Keeping blood sugar steady; supplying your body with the raw materials it needs to manufacture hormones; and creating a calm, relaxed environment for eating and digesting are all at the core of hormone health. The following diet suggestions will set you on the path to hormone balance and abundant health and beauty.

- Don't believe that low-fat/no-fat foods are best. Good fats like avocado, flaxseed oil, coconut oil, raw nuts, seeds, olive oil, cold-water fish, and chia seeds are essential for hormone production. The essential fats in many of these foods also help to balance and stabilize hormones and lower cortisol. And while you're incorporating good fats, eliminate Beauty Betrayers, in the form of fried or processed foods that most likely contain trans fats, which can aggravate, even cause, a hormonal imbalance.

- Eat organic. The fewer pesticides and additives that your body has to contend with, the more energy it has to keep your hormones happy.

- Eat adequate protein to keep your blood sugar from rapidly rising and falling. Eat Pretty sources include wild salmon and sardines, pastured eggs, spirulina, raw nuts, and hemp seeds.

- Crunch cruciferous vegetables, which assist in the elimination of excess estrogens, thanks to a phytochemical called indole-3-carbinol. Some of the most powerful cruciferous veggies are kale, cabbage, Brussels sprouts, broccoli, bok choy, and cauliflower.

- Choose foods that nourish your hormone-producing adrenal glands, including sea vegetables like nori, dulse, and kombu (consult your doctor, however, if you have thyroid issues that may be affected by iodine-rich foods); and beans, including kidney and black beans.

- Limit refined sugar and processed foods to lower inflammation and stabilize insulin spikes. Don't forget, alcohol is also a sugar, and it increases estrogen in women and men alike.

- If you consume dairy and meat, choose only high-quality hormone-free sources. Conventional milk has added hormones that stimulate acne-causing androgens in the body.

- Vitamin C–rich foods like raw bell peppers, citrus fruits, broccoli, and leafy greens may actually curb stress by lowering the amount of cortisol released by your body.

- Stay hydrated. Dehydration causes your body to release cortisol and histamines. The result is blood acidity, and a decrease in the amount of oxygen your red blood cells take in.

- Dark chocolate (at least 70 percent cacao, and in moderation) can lower blood pressure and give your brain an endorphin surge that's mood enhancing. And there's the hope that dark chocolate might hold even greater powers: one study found that just over 1 oz/30 g of dark chocolate daily could mediate the metabolic effects of stress and lower cortisol levels.

- Skip coffee, since it stimulates cortisol production (green tea is still okay for a touch of caffeine and a blast of antioxidants). Instead, sip chamomile tea to calm the body and decrease anxiety, or tulsi tea (see page 128) to support your body's ability to manage stress.

Breathe

Breathing—for beauty? Trust me when I say that no one approached the connection between beauty, hormones, and breath with greater skepticism than myself. Could a practice as simple as mindful breathing make a measurable difference in the body? Consider this: each breath brings vital oxygen to our bodily tissues, removes acidic carbon dioxide waste, and encourages nutrient delivery to our cells through healthy circulation. Oxygen is essential for the production of ATP, which circulates energy in the body.

I ignored the message about the value of breathing exercises for years before I eked out a place for mindful breath in my own daily routine. When I finally immersed myself in the practice, the calming, energizing results were remarkable. Breathing happens to be one of the few things you actually *don't* have to think about, so I'll admit it's kind of a shame to have to add it to your to-do list. But bringing awareness to your breath is a gift to yourself.

So many of us take in only short, shallow breaths, and miss out on precious energy and waste removal for our cells. We allow our stress levels to rise and rise, unchecked. Our beauty is missing out! Try this basic breathing for beauty plan today: take several deep, deliberate breaths from your diaphragm when you wake in the morning, before each meal, before you go to bed at night, and at any other time when you remember: sitting on the subway, in the bathroom, or doing chores (every breath counts!). Stop and breathe in deeply through your nose right now. Don't you feel fuller, calmer, more nourished already?

Work It Out

As you now know, if you don't let your stress hormones get out of control, they aren't around to crash the healthy hormone party. Let's change the belief that chronic stress is an inevitable part of our lives. I challenge you to come up with your own personal de-stressing routine, and tailor it to your daily needs. This means mixing up cardio and strength training with calming exercises in your workout routine, according to the state of your health and your stress level. Just got your period and finished an intense strategy session at the office? A long walk or restorative yoga session is in order. Woke up earlier than normal on a beautiful morning? Squeeze in an extra-long run with a few powerful sprints, or take a high-intensity spinning class. Been sitting at the office all day? Try dancing to your favorite songs for thirty minutes to boost your mood and lower cortisol.

Find stress relief, and beauty, in creativity, and do not underestimate the power of escaping to nature. One study found that walking in nature decreased cortisol levels by 12.4 percent, compared to an urban environment. Overall you want to be sure your workouts relieve stress, rather than compound it. For many of us, overexercising aggravates hormone imbalance. More is not necessarily more, especially if it causes stress and strain on our bodies.

Massage

Have you ever noticed that, in addition to the tension release, you just seem to sparkle the day after a massage? I'm sure I don't need to remind you what a little hands-on touch can do for your stress level, or your appearance. The overwhelming sense of calm and well-being that you get from a good massage isn't in your head—in fact, one study found that a forty-five-minute Swedish massage gives the body a measurable health and beauty boost by decreasing cortisol and increasing circulating lymphocytes, which suggests that you walk away from a rub-down with both a mood lift *and* an immune boost.

Massage also revs up the flow of lymph, the fluid that circulates in the body just under the skin, carrying nutrients and filtering toxins. Stagnant lymph can cause many of the same symptoms as a hormonal imbalance, so support lymph flow with either a massage or dry brushing session.

I've experienced great calming, hormone-balancing benefits from the traditional Eastern practice of self-massage. To do a self-massage at home, slightly warm some natural, fragrance-free oil like coconut or sesame and take 5 minutes or more to massage it into your body, starting at the ends of your limbs and working inward toward your heart. Massage your stomach in a clockwise motion. Finally, shower to rinse your skin, but try not to wash away all of the oil. As any skin care expert will tell you, oiling up the body also keeps skin supple and hydrated, so you'll enjoy twice the beautifying effects.

Shop Smart

It breaks my heart to tell beauty lovers everywhere that so many of the products they consider to be the most beautifying have a fiercely ugly side: they exacerbate hormonal issues. There is nothing beautiful about ingredients like parabens, phthalates, and synthetic fragrance, common in conventional beauty products, all of which are known to disrupt the natural function of your endocrine system. I encourage you to look closely at the ingredients in your personal care products before you buy them or apply them to your skin. The less demand there is for these toxic products, the less they will be produced—and end up contaminating our bodies and environment. Think of natural and organic personal care as an extension of your Eat Pretty lifestyle. You already know that feeding your beauty from the inside does wonders for your skin, and it only makes sense that your *topical* skin diet (after all, your skin absorbs 60 percent of the products you apply) would match it in quality.

Limiting your exposure to chemicals from pesticides, plastics, cleaning supplies, and beauty products, many of which behave like estrogens in the body—we call these synthetic imposters xenoestrogens—is a critical way to support your body's hormone balance. The chemicals you put on your body today can and will affect you now and in later years. Xenoestrogens have wide-ranging health effects, from triggering early puberty in girls and problems with male reproductive organs to altering the signaling of thyroid hormones. And a recent study suggests that xenoestrogens in beauty products and processed foods could cause early menopause in women as young as their mid-thirties. They're also thought to accumulate in fat and possibly contribute to cellulite.

You might think that any beauty product available on store shelves would be safe to use, but plenty of ingredients in our products are untested. Make sure that the skincare formulas you choose are clean enough to eat. It's a confusing time in the beauty industry, so it helps to be loyal to brands and retailers you trust, at least until consumers are better protected. You won't need a boatload of products (after all, your diet and lifestyle are laying a radiant foundation), but a lineup of quality beauty essentials is a major asset. Some products, like sunscreen, are constantly evolving, so look for the newest natural advances (see Resources, page 200).

Believe it or not, nasty hormone disruptors show up in plenty of other places around your home. Switch to natural cleaning products (baking soda and vinegar are multitasking heroes—try them!), limit your exposure to toxic dry-cleaning chemicals, and throw away—or don't buy—plastics labeled 3, 6, or 7, which pose health risks for their levels of BPA and other chemicals that compromise hormone health. Store your leftovers in glass containers; they're far prettier, and are also perfect for serving and reheating. The fewer chemicals you take in, the more your fabulous body can focus on keeping you hormonally healthy, and gorgeous.

If you think about it, all of this is actually an incredibly luxurious prescription, one that fits in with the core message of the Eat Pretty lifestyle. Really, when was the last time you let go of other obligations to take the time and space to breathe deeply, or massaged your body head to toe with organic oils? Hormone balance, like healthy beauty, is rooted in self-love. It's time to give yourself the pampering you need to be your healthiest, happiest, and most beautiful, so that you can share your gifts with others. It's about more than simply deserving it. Understanding your hormones and correcting imbalances now can prevent chronic health issues like cancer, diabetes, heart disease, and Alzheimer's later in life. This prescription for healthy hormones goes on the top of your to-do list; give it priority over errands and deadlines. In doing so, you'll honor your healthy vanity.

Plastics 3, 6, 7 BPA

BEAUTY SLEEP

You know you look better when you sleep well, but do you actually eat better when you sleep well, too? You're about to witness the beautifying cycle of sleep: Eat Pretty foods and habits help you max out the beauty benefits of sleep, and those restful hours make it easier to maintain your Eat Pretty diet during every waking moment.

Eat Pretty for Beautiful Sleep

Picture this: You walk into the office with a pounding head and collapse into your desk chair. Your eyes burn, your head is foggy, and you feel short-tempered even before the phone starts ringing. On your way to the kitchen for a second coffee (oh, there are *donuts!*) you catch a glimpse of yourself and realize that your skin is dull, and that your concealer doesn't begin to camouflage the bags under your eyes today. Your pants feel tighter than they did a week ago. If only you'd been able to fall asleep last night.

We've all felt something similar after a restless night, an all-nighter, or a long flight that disrupts our sleep schedule. Lack of sleep starts a cycle of un-pretty decisions and moods for the remainder of the day. If you did catch a full eight hours of rest, your day might start a little more like this: You walk into the office feeling confident in a figure-hugging dress topped with a fitted blazer—you feel slimmer today. Your morning mug of warm lemon water hydrated you, and now you're ready for breakfast, so you dive into the green smoothie that you made on your way out the door. Each sip is like a breath of fresh air for your cells, and it leaves your mind feel clear and focused. You launch right into the project you've been working on without hearing the constant call of the vending machine. Before lunch you stop in the bathroom to reapply lipstick and notice that your skin and eyes are shining. Those extra hours of rest were no joke!

The lesson: Don't mess with beauty sleep. Money won't buy it, you can't delegate it to your assistant, and you'd better not blow it off if you want to look and feel your best. Sleep shaves years off your appearance when you do it well and throws a wrench in your Eat Pretty lifestyle when you don't. It's a message you've probably heard before, one that science has underscored of late, with findings like a direct link between attractiveness and the number of hours slept. Study participants (who were already youthful, between eighteen and thirty-one) were judged to look 19 percent more tired, 6 percent less healthy, and 4 percent less attractive after just one night of reduced sleep. Our brains recognize symmetry and other signs of health and youth as measures of facial beauty, so your peers read your dark circles, puffiness, and sallow complexion after a rough night as un-pretty and unhealthy. Another study found that sleeping only four hours made participants less attractive and less *approachable* to their peers. Don't be surprised if your colleagues avoid you because you stayed up too late in the throes of a movie marathon!

Why don't we all just pencil in eight hours between dinner and breakfast? A regular sleep schedule is a cherished time out for some, but a major frustration for others. If you're one of the latter beauties who can't seem to make peace with pillow time, I want a sleep tune-up to be your top priority. If you don't sleep soundly, you're also not alone. It's not clear what causes the majority of our sleep disturbances, but stress, Beauty Betrayer foods, sleep environment, and technology are all definite factors. Without a night of *good* sleep, you're missing out on a rare treasure—free antiaging from within. You're adding unnecessary stress to your body and probably packing on unwanted pounds. Let's stop this chain of events before it ages your body and beauty much faster than you can control.

A night of quality sleep is worth a hundred eye creams. But what exactly makes sleep such a powerful beauty freebie? In more ways than one, the most attractive perk of a healthy sleep schedule could be a little something called human growth hormone, or HGH. The antiaging effects of growth hormone—a boost in skin cell production and collagen synthesis, and damage-reversing skin repair and rejuvenation—make it worth hitting the sack early. Growth hormone is a powerful way to hit rewind on some of the oxidative damage that occurs during an average day. The most important hour of sleep for growth hormone release turns out to be the very first hour (though the benefits increase if you make time for a full eight to nine hours), since you actually get more *deep* sleep toward the beginning of the night, and that's when the most growth hormone is secreted. Both deep sleep and growth hormone decline with age, so max out the beauty benefits while you can!

In case you were wondering, skipping your zzz's will not only fail to antiage you, it will prematurely age you. Instead of the drop in stress hormones that you experience while you snooze, lack of sleep adds fuel to the stressed-out fire with additional cortisol, which breaks down collagen and impairs the function of the skin barrier. Sleep deprivation also suppresses the immune system and creates inflammation in the body, which contributes to acne, rashes, wrinkles, redness, and dry skin. And you certainly won't *feel* your best, since sleep deprivation makes you depressed, moody, and anxious. Sleep takes the stress off your delicate adrenal glands, making it a powerful tool for preventing and healing adrenal fatigue. And recent studies have found that a good night of sleep increases the happy memories and positive images that we remember, while sleep deprivation can make us anxious, forgetful, and less grateful toward others.

The next best reason to tune up your sleep habits? The size of your waistline. Sleeping less than six hours, which many of us do routinely, is called partial sleep deprivation, and it has a major influence on the way we gain and lose weight. In general, sleep and weight are inversely related: more sleep means that we hold onto less weight, and less sleep equals more unwanted pounds.

Here's how it all goes down: First, lack of sleep raises the stress hormone cortisol in your body, making you crave comfort foods. You're more drawn to starchy, carby, sugary, and instantly gratifying Beauty Betrayers (like the donuts in your office kitchen). Too little sleep increases the likelihood that you'll overdo it on calories during the day, and it can decrease insulin sensitivity in your cells by as much as 30 percent. Lack of sleep also makes it harder for you to make smart decisions, so you're more likely to impulsively grab a candy bar from the vending machine without thinking about the Eat Pretty foods you brought from home. It's not your fault; your brain made you do it!

One study found that pictures of unhealthy foods activated reward signals in the brains of sleep-deprived participants. And guess what: the healthy foods didn't make those same bells ring. See how lack of sleep gets in the way of Eat Pretty choices? Too little sleep also causes hormonal changes that decrease your satiety after eating, lower the calories you burn during the day, and turn on obesity-promoting genes. No surprise that it's so easy to pack on the pounds when you don't sleep well. Time to find out how to get your beauty sleep back.

What's Keeping You Awake?

Sleep is a powerful beauty tool! Lack of sleep can mess with your moods, your food cravings, and even bring on a breakout by increasing your levels of cortisol, the stress hormone that causes inflammation and turns on your oil-producing glands. For a major beauty boost, watch out for the following sneaky sleep saboteurs.

Technology

Melatonin, a hormone emitted as you settle down to sleep, gets confused by the blue light coming from your laptop, smartphone, TV—you name it. Cue a flashback of the last time you checked Facebook in bed, in the dark. Staring into any of these devices within an hour of bedtime can seriously disrupt your sleep. In general, keep them out of the bedroom. If you have trouble falling asleep nightly, talk to your doctor about a melatonin supplement.

Diet

You already know that an afternoon coffee can keep you from restful sleep, but what about a late dinner? Chowing down (especially on a heavy, hard-to-digest meal) within two hours of bedtime steals energy that should be devoted to rest and repair and puts it toward digestive duties. Digestion also raises your internal body temperature at a time of day when your temperature should be dropping to signal bedtime.

If you're hungry before bed, a small snack is okay, even beneficial, as long as you choose wisely. Go for beauty foods that contain calming minerals like magnesium and potassium (bananas, which are easy on the digestive system, contain both), calcium (warm almond milk with a little nutmeg is an ideal sleep drink), or a bit of protein, specifically protein that contains the amino acid tryptophan to help your body manufacture serotonin, the neurotransmitter that calms and relaxes. Pumpkin seeds, millet, and naturally smoked wild salmon are good choices. Tart cherry juice also enhances melatonin production, so a few sips before bed can promote restful sleep. Stay away from dark chocolate or sugary foods that leave you jittery and wired.

If you are used to eating several small daily meals or grazing all day long, you might wake up after a few hours of sleep because of low blood sugar. In this case, you can try to space out your meals and eat a small protein-rich snack before bed to keep your blood sugar steady. During the day, make sure you get adequate B vitamins, which aid in serotonin production, and vitamin D, which reduces daytime sleepiness. And skip the nightcap. Even though it relaxes you initially, alcohol before bed can also interfere with sleep, since it disrupts the deep sleep and REM sleep that are essential for maximum beauty benefits.

Environment

Your sleep spot should be rather cave-like: cool, dark, and quiet. It's best to keep your bedroom completely dark at night, but not so blacked out that you miss the natural wake-up progression of the sun. And maintain a comfortable sleep temperature, between 55 and 75°F/13 and 24°C.

Stress

Had just about enough of work worries interrupting your beauty sleep? You're not alone. They're not worth the loss of precious shut-eye. Whether your brain can't turn off its worry circuit or your mind speeds up as soon as your head hits the pillow, creating a nighttime ritual can help you settle into sleep mode. Leave your stress at the bedroom door by taking time to discharge your thoughts in a journal a few hours before bed. Write down your worries, unresolved problems, and tomorrow's to-do list, and leave it outside your bedroom, where you can pick it up tomorrow.

Pamper Your Way to the Pillow

Comfy mattress, clean sheets, maybe a little lavender in the air—there are plenty of ways to set the stage for antiaging sleep. Here are my absolute favorite rituals to prepare your body for a night of beautifying rest:

Soaking

A warm bath before bed raises your core body temperature, which then dips when you leave the water, signaling to your brain that it's time to sleep. Your body temperature naturally cools before bed, and soaking naturally mimics the process by raising your temperature enough that your body relaxes, your stress releases, and your cortisol lowers as you cool to a normal temperature.

Breathing

Meditation or mindful breathing before bed is a good way to create total-body relaxation that prepares you for sleep. Just ten minutes of meditation or deep breathing can promote deep calm, and it may even put you to sleep. One study actually found that mindfulness-based meditation had sleep-inducing effects similar to that of a popular sleep aid—without the side effects, of course. To start a simple meditation practice, sit upright in a comfortable position. Close your eyes, clear your head of thoughts and worries, and concentrate only on the deep inward (through your nose) and outward (through your mouth) flow of your breath. If your mind drifts, let go of your thoughts once more and return to focus on your breathing. Sit for at least five and up to ten minutes at first. Work up to a longer session, if you desire.

Sipping

Before bed, try a cup of herbal tea (chamomile, rooibos, and lavender are good picks), which raises and lowers your core temperature in a manner similar to a bath. Another sleep-inducing sip: a powdered magnesium supplement that you stir into hot water (see Resources, page 200). Magnesium relaxes muscles and creates a feeling of calm before bed.

Stretching

A small study of twenty people with insomnia found that daily yoga practice helped participants fall asleep significantly faster, and sleep better and longer. Regular aerobic exercise will also increase deep sleep and growth hormone, not to mention its circulatory benefits for the skin—just finish aerobic exercise at least four hours before bed.

Feel the Rhythm

One more reason that sleep is so powerful for your beauty is its influence over your body clock, the circadian rhythms that guide metabolic processes, appetite, body temperature, and even mood. Sleep synchronizes so many of the processes that relate to your beauty and body. Waking up at the same time each day can help keep your circadian rhythms in check. Even if you hit the sack a few hours late, it helps to get up relatively close to your normal wake-up time.

Still, your sleep habits will change through new periods in your life and with the seasons. Winter is the time to go to bed earlier and rest and rejuvenate your beauty, while summer, with its light evenings, could prompt a later bedtime. Generally speaking, you need seven to nine hours of sleep, but about 1 percent of the population are outliers who need as little as six or as much as ten hours. If you wake up tired every day you might be one of those people who needs more beauty sleep. To measure your optimal sleeping time, see how many hours you sleep when you are on vacation and can wake up without an alarm. Now, try to get vacation-length beauty sleep every night when you're back at home!

MIND AND MOVEMENT

Stress and emotions play a major role in a lifetime of good looks. To amplify the benefits of your Eat Pretty foods, support your emotional health with the mind-body tools I've outlined in the pages ahead. They offer even more ways to glow from the inside out.

Eat Pretty for Beautiful Moods

Turning beauty inside out means looking at the influence of your mind, as well as your body, on your appearance. Look closely and you'll find that you need more than just physical nourishment to foster your best self. The Eat Pretty foods on your plate are the foundation of your beauty and body—and they're also essential elements of your mental well-being. But food alone can't sustain the happiness, calm, mindfulness, and joy needed for your most beautiful life. Those emotions thrive with attention and self-care.

If you've ever struggled with a beauty issue that you felt powerless to change, you know that emotional health has strong ties to the skin, the hair, and the body you see in the mirror. Your emotions not only influence the way you see yourself, casting a positive or negative light, they have a physiological connection to your skin. The brain and skin both originate from the same part of the embryo, called the ectoderm, linking these two organs before we even enter the world.

But you don't need to study the development of our bodies to appreciate the brain-beauty link. If you've ever felt your cheeks flush with embarrassment, noticed extra sparkle when you're in love, or dealt with an outbreak of pimples or a rash while you're under stress, you know it exists. Your brain prompts the release of neuropeptides in your skin that can cause an increase in inflammation or a boost in sebum production that leads to a breakout. Our nervous system also controls sweating, the oil glands in our skin, the dilation of our blood vessels, even goosebumps that cause our hair to stand on end. Some people wear their heart on their sleeve, but we all wear our emotions on our epidermis, whether we like it or not.

Certainly sustained emotions like stress and depression make the most noticeable changes in our looks. Those emotions also have the most scientific study supporting their connection to beauty and health. Recent studies show that not only do males perceive females with high levels of the stress hormone cortisol to be less attractive, but women often have the same tendency, viewing guys with lower cortisol as the more appealing mates. Still not convinced that you can truly think and feel yourself pretty? For more proof of the powerful influence of your mind over your body, just look at the negative effects that stress has on your appearance. Stress:

- boosts inflammation.
- increases muscle tension, restricting blood flow to your tissues.
- releases cortisol, which breaks down collagen in the skin.
- hastens breathing, lowering oxygen intake and waste removal.

- causes and/or aggravates acne.
- contributes to dryness and sensitive skin.
- slows cell turnover and new skin cell production.
- impedes digestion and assimilation of beauty nutrients.
- increases cravings for un-pretty foods.
- creates free radicals and damages DNA.
- aggravates dermatitis and psoriasis.
- thins skin and accelerates wrinkling.
- triggers adrenaline and therefore histamines, which can lead to hives and rashes.
- can precipitate hair loss.
- increases susceptibility to bacterial skin infections.
- promotes abdominal weight gain.
- lowers immunity.

All of this, from a state of mind that most of us experience daily? Witnessing the effects of stress on your appearance only serves to increase the stress burden and worsen the cycle. And stress isn't the only emotion that messes with our beauty (cue the furrow lines): one interesting study on the brain-beauty connection found that participants with low levels of anger control were more likely to exhibit delayed healing from a skin wound. Another study found that participants who watched a distressing movie clip reported significantly more pain and itch in their skin than those who watched a happy clip. Noticing skin issues when you're under emotional strain isn't in your mind after all. Still, I believe that increasing joy, pleasure, and relaxation is equally as influential in deepening overall beauty as reducing stress and anger. Boosting these positive emotions reduces inflammation and strengthens the type of beauty you want to build with Eat Pretty.

From a Western perspective, our state of mind doesn't factor strongly in the way we look day to day. Sure, you've been encouraged to "think positive," but it's always been an apple a day that kept the doctor away, not a meditation session. But that isn't the whole story. I think our perspective on emotional health is about to undergo a serious shift, similar to our new appreciation of beauty from within. Your mind has power over your beauty and health that can't be overstated. Just think: beauty could hinge just as much on the way you *feel* about your haircut as the way your hair actually looks today.

But here's where I can see a roadblock: we are prone to self-criticism. Healthy vanity requires self-acceptance and self-love! We've exposed the smoke and mirrors involved in fashion and beauty photography (some beauty product ads have now been banned around the world for misleading digital enhancements), but we still hold ourselves to unrealistic ideals. Certainly that undue stress and self-criticism isn't helping us to look and feel any more beautiful. If we are going to build beauty on a deeper level, we need to accept that we were born beautiful. A negative, self-critical mindset truly steals from our beauty. It trickles down into other aspects of our lives, and takes away joy that we might otherwise experience. Self-criticism and self-doubt are like toxins for your beauty.

Find Beauty in Self-Love

Happiness? Peace? Self-esteem? Whatever you call it, you can boost your emotional well-being with a dose of self-love. Start with these beautifying techniques:

Appreciation and Intention

For just a moment, appreciate yourself for devoting precious energy to the quality of your beauty and health. When you expressed the desire to deepen your beauty and health—and acted on it—you proved yourself to be exceptional. In the midst of your busy life, you're choosing to support and love *you*. No one else can make that choice that for you.

Throughout Part 2 of this book, I offered advice for how to set seasonal intentions for deepening your beauty. Intentions are very powerful tools in your Eat Pretty lifestyle. I also want you to set the intention to do one kind thing for yourself every day, no matter what the season.

Give yourself an extra half an hour of sleep; buy yourself a bouquet of flowers; make time for a quiet walk. Small expressions of self-love and gratitude like these reinforce your value, and they help you develop an appreciation for your body. They also restore feelings of accomplishment, positivity, and confidence. Can't you already feel the immense power you have over your lifestyle of beauty? You have that power over your happiness as well. Practice setting intentions for yourself in the short and the long term, and use them to appreciate every step of your Eat Pretty journey. You'll find that the energy rubs off in many other areas of life as well.

Breathing and Meditation

What's weighing on your mind at this very moment? What emotional burden stresses you or makes you angry today? Whatever it is, it's holding back your beauty. Rather than seek out a (possibly nonexistent) solution to your worry, your goal is to release its hold on your beauty using the science-backed power of your breath and your mind. We all experience stress or sadness or anger at times, so it is truly our ability to fall back in to a safe, calm space that allows us to conquer negative emotions and build beauty and security. Two of our greatest tools are breathing and meditation (see page 190 for meditation instructions).

Managing stress and anxiety is one of my greatest beauty challenges. I held out for ages before I made time to take deep, meaningful breaths and clear my mind with moments of meditation. The beauty benefits are many: deep breathing relaxes your facial muscles and boosts circulation of fresh oxygen and nutrients within your body. It even rids the body of toxins several times faster than normal breath.

Remember, the feeling of well-being you get from meditation is not all in your head: meditation is a proven antiaging practice for your body. It only follows that your beauty benefits as well. I believe that the power of meditation lies in its ability to offer a sense of control, at the same time lessening your need to maintain such tight control over your life.

Recent studies suggest there's even more to it. In one study, researchers linked both stress and *perceptions* of stress to our telomeres, which are the protective end caps of our chromosomes. Shortened telomeres—which are signs of physical aging—were associated with high stress levels. Another study found a link between meditation and the reduced activation of aging, inflammatory genes. Proof that your mind is a strong protector of beauty and youth.

Mood Food

Eat Pretty creates pampering through beauty nutrition. Those amazing beauty foods for skin, hair, and nails also contain the building blocks for the neurotransmitters that profoundly influence your brain chemistry. Brain chemicals are critical to feeling satiated, happy, and focused. The proteins and fats necessary to building healthy brain chemicals also balance your blood sugar, which directly affects your mood throughout the day (not just when you're over-hungry). The wrong food choices take you on a blood sugar roller coaster and can actually make you feel sad, anxious, depressed, and unhappy with your beauty.

The foods that promote brain health (and also happen to feed your skin) are complex carbs, healthy fats, and proteins like wild salmon, sardines, raw nuts and seeds, quinoa, lentils, avocados, ground flaxseed, and olive oil—Eat Pretty foods that you already stock in your pantry. Abundant seasonal beauty veggies and fruits are also key. Eating seven portions of fruit and vegetables a day has been shown to increase happiness and mental health. Alternatively, a diet high in processed foods has been linked to a higher risk of depression compared to a diet rich in whole foods. An overload of Beauty Betrayers like sugar, processed foods, and alcohol can diminish the number of dopamine (pleasure) receptors in your brain, so by eating them regularly you're negatively altering your brain function. What happens? You continue to need more of those processed foods to feel satisfied.

Eating those Beauty Betrayer foods also sets you up for emotional eating. We often blame a rough day or a bad breakup for our tendency to overindulge and feel out of control in our eating habits, but sometimes we're just reacting to the foods we've been eating that leave our bodies emotionally imbalanced. Foods like refined sugars, simple carbs, caffeinated sodas and coffee, processed fats—even pesticide-laden produce, since pesticides can be neurotoxic—negatively influence our emotional health.

Move Your Body, Make Over Your Mind

When you see exercise as a tool for beauty and happiness, rather than a task to check off your to-do list, you have a big reason to *want* it. That's just one more secret to maintaining an Eat Pretty lifestyle. Plenty of us exercise to look good in a bikini, which can be an absolutely healthy goal, but if this goal creates too much pressure, your emotional health can take a hit. It's important to make sure you exercise for *you*.

Here's why you should break a sweat today: exercise increases circulation that brings fresh nutrition to your cells, and it revs up lymph flow for extra detoxification, lessening the burden on your skin. Weight-bearing exercises keep your bones strong, while exercise of all kinds reduces inflammation and stress, in part because of the feel-good release of endorphins (they give you a radiant post-workout glow) and the neurotransmitters serotonin and dopamine. One study found that women who exercised three hours a week had a 30 percent lower chance of developing psoriasis (a condition linked to inflammation) compared to those who didn't exercise at all.

Exercise not only burns calories, but helps regulate appetite and fullness, thanks to a specific protein secreted by muscles when they contract. Breaking a sweat also gives you an immune boost for about three hours after a workout. Two interesting ways to max out the beauty and health benefits of your workout: exercise with a friend, which can raise your pain threshold so you put a little more effort into your routine; and take it outdoors, where fresh air and a fresh view may boost mood and self-esteem (even if it's only five minutes).

For an even bigger boost, head to water, like a lake, river, or the beach. The most surprising news about working out? More is not necessarily better. In a recent study, participants exercising for thirty minutes daily lost just as much weight as those exercising an hour a day. Another recent study of women over sixty found that working out just twice a week resulted in boosts in energy and fitness comparable to those gained by working out four and six times a week. Too much exercise stresses your body and can make your routine difficult to maintain. So find that just-right balance. Unless you're training for a specific event or goal, don't get tunnel vision on exercise. Mix it up, keep it fun, alternate indoor classes with outdoor jogs and yoga with strength training. And know when to stay home and rest. The effects of overtraining (you've seen them on a few celebs) can be just as aging as no exercise at all.

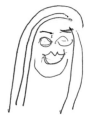

❯❯ CONTINUING YOUR EAT PRETTY JOURNEY ❮❮

Take this moment to look at yourself—already healthier, wiser, and more gorgeous than ever before. You now have a rich collection of tools to support your lifestyle of beauty from the inside, tools that you might not have known about yesterday. Be kind to yourself as you start a lifestyle that may feel very new. Practice listening to your body's needs. And always lean on your foundation—fresh, seasonal Eat Pretty foods—to see you over beauty bumps in the road. They'll always be available to help you look and feel your most beautiful.

Above all, enjoy your unique Eat Pretty journey! Try unfamiliar beauty foods and experiment with new recipes. Taste, smell, see, and savor the beauty in your food. Discover a brand new way to feel pampered, even as you make over your beauty and body one molecule at a time. Remember, eating for beauty is a powerful tool that is accessible to us all, but not many know how to use it. You are one of those special few who understand the inside-out approach to beauty. You can share your knowledge and your radiant glow with everyone in your life. I wish you a lifetime of looking and feeling your best, and years filled with the beauty of Eat Pretty.

Beauty Is Wellness
www.beautyiswellness.com

For the most up-to-date beauty and health news, beautifying recipes, natural products, and daily inspiration to maintain your Eat Pretty lifestyle, Beauty Is Wellness is Jolene's home online. Visit the site to arrange an in-person or remote coaching session or cooking class with Jolene, and to find out about workshops, online programs, and new publications.

Recommended Books

Absolute Beauty, by Pratima Raichur (HarperCollins, 1997).

Balance Your Hormones, Balance Your Life, by Claudia Welch, MSOM (Da Capo Press, 2011).

The Beauty Detox Solution, by Kimberly Snyder, C.N. (Harlequin, 2011).

The Beauty Diet, by Lisa Drayer, M.A., R.D. (McGraw-Hill, 2009).

Feed Your Face, by Jessica Wu, M.D. (St. Martin's Press, 2011).

Food and Healing, by Annemarie Colbin (Random House, 1986).

Forever Young, by Nicholas Perricone, M.D. (Atria Books, 2010).

The Gorgeously Green Diet, by Sophie Uliano (Penguin Group, 2009).

The Green Beauty Guide, by Julie Gabriel (Health Communications, 2008).

Healing with Whole Foods, by Paul Pitchford (North Atlantic Books, 1993).

The Living Beauty Detox Program, by Ann Louise Gittleman, M.S., C.N.S. (HarperCollins, 2000).

No More Dirty Looks, by Siobhan O'Connor and Alexandra Spunt (Da Capo Press, 2010).

Stop Aging, Start Living, by Jeannette Graf, M.D. (Three Rivers Press, 2007).

Wheat Belly, by William Davis, M.D. (Rodale, 2011).

WomanCode, by Alisa Vitti (HarperCollins, 2013).

Informational Websites

Dr. Frank Lipman *www.drfranklipman.com*

Environmental Working Group's Cosmetics Database and Sunscreen Guide *www.ewg.org/skindeep*

FloLiving *floliving.com*

Gorgeously Green
www.gorgeouslygreen.com

Institute for Integrative Nutrition
www.integrativenutrition.com

LifeSpa *lifespa.com*

Natural Gourmet Institute
www.naturalgourmetinstitute.com

Nutrition Data *nutritiondata.self.com*

Personalized Lifestyle Medicine
Institute *www.plminstitute.org*

PubMed *www.pubmed.gov*

Online Natural Beauty Retailers

Beautorium *www.beautorium.com*

NuboNau *nubonau.com*

O&N Collective *oandncollective.com*

Saffron Rouge *www.saffronrouge.com*

Spirit Beauty Lounge
www.spiritbeautylounge.com

Natural Product Sources

BROAD-SPECTRUM NATURAL SUNSCREENS

Badger *www.badgerbalm.com*

Coola *www.coolasuncare.com*

MyChelle *www.mychelle.com*

True Natural *www.truenatural.com*

NATURAL AND ORGANIC FRAGRANCES

Honoré Des Prés *honoredespres.com*

La Bella Figura *labellafigurabeauty.com*

Strange Invisible Perfumes
www.siperfumes.com

Tata Harper
www.tataharperskincare.com

Tsi-La Organics *tsilaorganics.com*

NATURAL DEODORANTS

Bubble and Bee *www.bubbleandbee.com*

Nourish Organic *nourishorganic.com*

Soapwalla *soapwallakitchen.com*

Weleda *www.weleda.com*

KITCHEN AND HEALTH TOOLS

Floradix iron supplement
www.floradix.net

Natural Calm magnesium supplement
www.naturalvitality.com

Vitamix blender *www.vitamix.com*

TEA

Kusmi Tea *kusmitea.com*

Mountain Rose Herbs
mountainroseherbs.com

Organic India *organicindia.com*

Pukka *www.pukkaherbs.com*

Traditional Medicinals
www.traditionalmedicinals.com

ACKNOWLEDGMENTS

Many special people contributed to the writing of this book, whether by word, deed, or presence in my life. I am deeply grateful to every one of you.

Especially to Megan Sovern, my literary matchmaker, for your confidence in my message, your determination to make it heard—and for leading by example.

To Elizabeth Yarborough, my brilliant editor, steadfast cheerleader, and intermittent therapist. I couldn't be happier to have you as my guide on this amazing journey.

To the entire Chronicle Books team for seeing the beauty in *Eat Pretty* from the very beginning. Thank you for bringing my passion to print.

My sincere gratitude goes to the estimable experts who informed, inspired, and supported the writing of this book: Catherine Darley, John Douillard, Jeannette Graf, Frank Lipman, Deanna Minich, Joanna Vargas, Alisa Vitti, and Claudia Welch. Thank you for so generously giving of your time and your knowledge. To the other thought leaders who influenced my beauty journey: Nicholas Perricone, Ann Louise Gittleman, Sophie Uliano, Rosemary Gladstar, and Pratima Raichur.

To beauty and wellness gurus Jane Iredale, Lina Hanson, Ewa Asmar, Tata Harper, Miranda Kerr, and Sophie for imparting your words of wisdom for a beautiful life.

To Amanda, Megan, Meghan, Laura, and Alexis for your thoughtful notes on my proposal when *Eat Pretty* was just beginning to take shape. To Marietta and Rona, for sharing your knowledge with a first-timer.

To my family and friends for surrounding me with endless love and support, even (and especially) when I work too much. And to Rob, for being a tireless champion of my talent and my dreams, and reminding me that with love, anything is possible.

Chapter 1: Beauty Betrayers

p. 17, regarding milk consumption causing a rise in oil-producing hormones in adults: "Role of insulin, insulin-like growth factor-1, hyperglycaemic food and milk consumption in the pathogenesis of acne vulgaris," *Experimental Dermatology*, August 2009.

p. 20, regarding phosphates in soda being linked to skin atrophy: "Dietary evidence for phosphate toxicity accelerating mammalian aging," *Journal of the Federation of American Societies for Experimental Biology*, September 2010.

p. 22, regarding oxidative stress and gray hair: "Oxidative stress in ageing of hair," *International Journal of Trichology*, January 2009.

"Basic evidence for epidermal $H_2O_2/OONO^-$-mediated oxidation/nitration in segmental vitiligo is supported by repigmentation of skin and eyelashes after reduction of epidermal H_2O_2 with topical NB-UVB-activated pseudocatalase PC-KUS," *Journal of the Federation of American Societies for Experimental Biology*, April 2013.

p. 26, regarding dairy and sugar as contributors to breakouts: "Diet and acne: a review of the evidence," *International Journal of Dermatology*, April 2009.

p. 26, regarding how an increase in dietary fruit and vegetables makes skin look plumper and more hydrated: "An encapsulated fruit and vegetable juice concentrate increases skin microcirculation in healthy women," *Skin Pharmacology and Physiology*, August 2011.

p. 26, regarding how boosting veggie intake makes us more attractive to others: "You are what you eat: within-subject increases in fruit and vegetable consumption confer beneficial skin-color changes," PLOS One, March 2012.

Chapter 9: Beauty Beyond Your Plate

p. 164, regarding exploration of the human microbiome: "Structure, function and diversity of the healthy human microbiome," *Nature*, June 2012.

p. 165, regarding the study of the gut-brain-skin axis: "Acne vulgaris, probiotics, and the gut-brain-skin axis—back to the future?" *Gut Pathogens*, January 2011.

p. 165, regarding the link between tetracycline-class antibiotics and IBD: "Potential association between the oral tetracycline class of antimicrobials used to treat acne and inflammatory bowel disease," *American Journal of Gastroenterology*, December 2010.

p. 165, regarding the link between bacterial overgrowth and rosacea: "Small intestinal bacterial overgrowth in rosacea: clinical effectiveness of its eradication," *Clinical Gastroenterology and Hepatology*, July 2008.

p. 165, regarding the link between *H. pylori* bacteria and hives: "Possible benefit from treatment of *Helicobacter pylori* in antihistamine-resistant chronic urticaria," *Clinical and Experimental Dermatology*, January 2013.

p. 170, regarding evidence that coriander, mint, and lemon balm together alleviate IBS symptoms: "The efficacy of an herbal medicine, Carmint, on the relief of abdominal pain and bloating in patients with irritable bowel syndrome," *Digestive Diseases and Sciences*, August 2006.

p. 170, regarding how peppermint can ease gas, nausea, indigestion: *The Woman's Book of Healing Herbs*, Harrar, Sari and Sara Altshul O'Donnell, Rodale Press, 1999.

p. 171, regarding the link between *Saccharomyces boulardii* and acne: "Treatment of acne with a yeast preparation," *Fortschritte der Medizin* [German], September 1989.

p. 173, regarding how 44 percent of women struggle with hormonal breakouts: *Feed Your Face*, Wu, Jessica, St. Martin's Press, 2011.

p. 175, regarding the link between stress and skin reactivity and sensitivity: "Managing stress can help people improve their skin conditions," *American Academy of Dermatology* (aad.org), August 2011.

p. 176, regarding IGF-1 and large pores: "Serum levels of IGF-1 are related to human skin characteristics including the conspicuousness of facial pores," *International Journal of Cosmetic Science*, April 2011.

p. 177, regarding how stored fat acts as an endocrine organ: "Identification of novel human adipocyte secreted proteins by using SGBS cells," *Journal of Proteome Research*, August 2010.

p. 179, regarding evidence that Vitamin C–rich foods can lower cortisol levels: "Mood Food," Oz, Mehmet, *O, The Oprah Magazine*, November 2012.

p. 179, regarding evidence that dark chocolate mediates the effects of stress and lowers cortisol levels: "Metabolic effects of dark chocolate consumption on energy, gut microbiota, and stress-related metabolism in free-living subjects," *Journal of Proteome Research*, October 2009.

p. 181, regarding evidence that walking in nature decreases cortisol: "Preventative medical effects of nature therapy," *Japanese Journal of Hygiene*, September 2011.

p. 181, regarding the benefits of Swedish massage: "A preliminary study of the effects of a single session of Swedish massage on hypothalamic-pituitary-adrenal and immune function in normal individuals," *Journal of Alternative and Complementary Medicine*, September 2010.

p. 182, regarding evidence that xenoestrogens can cause early menopause: "Early Menopause: Study says Common Item Can Be a Trigger," Emling, Shelley, The Huffington Post (huffingtonpost.com), October 29, 2012.

p. 185, regarding the link between attractiveness and sleep: "Beauty sleep: experimental study on the perceived health and attractiveness of sleep deprived people," *British Medical Journal*, December 2010.

p. 185, regarding the link between sleep and approachability: "The effects of sleep restriction on attractiveness and social desirability," *21st Congress of the European Sleep Research Society*, September 2012.

p. 186, regarding sleep deprivation: "Processing of emotional reactivity and emotional memory over sleep," *Journal of Neuroscience*, January 2012.

p. 186, regarding partial sleep deprivation: "Partial Sleep Deprivation and Energy Balance in Adults: an Emerging Issue for Consideration by Dietetics Practitioners," *Journal of the Academy of Nutrition and Dietetics*, November 2012.

p. 187, regarding the link between lack of sleep and insulin sensitivity: "Impaired insulin signaling in human adipocytes after experimental sleep restriction: a randomized, crossover study," *Annals of Internal Medicine*, October 2012.

p. 187, regarding the link between sleep and decision making: "How the Brain Becomes Impaired by Sleep Deprivation Leading to Improper Food Choices," *Medical News Today*, June 2012.

p. 187, regarding how unhealthy food activates reward signals in the brain: "Junk food may be more appealing to tired brains," *Medical News Today*, June 2012.

p. 190, regarding mindfulness practices and sleep: "Mindfulness-based stress reduction versus pharmacotherapy for chronic primary insomnia: a randomized controlled clinical trial," *Explore*, March–April 2011.

p. 190, regarding yoga practice and sleep: "Treatment of chronic insomnia with yoga: a preliminary study with sleep-wake diaries," *Applied Psychophysiology and Biofeedback*, December 2004.

p. 192, regarding the link between cortisol and attractiveness in women: "Facial attractiveness is related to women's cortisol and body fat, but not with immune responsiveness," *Biology Letters*, May 2013.

p. 192, regarding the link between cortisol and attractiveness in men: "Evidence for the stress-linked immunocompetence handicap hypothesis in human male faces," *Proceedings of the Royal Society B*, August 2010.

p. 193, regarding the link between anger control and skin healing: "The influence of anger expression on wound healing," *Brain, Behavior and Immunity*, December 2007.

p. 193, regarding the link between movie clips and skin reactions: "Role of induced negative and positive emotions in sensitivity to itch and pain in women," *British Journal of Dermatology*, August 2012.

p. 196, regarding the link between stress and shortened telomeres: "Can meditation slow rate of cellular aging? Cognitive stress, mindfulness and telomeres," *Annals of the New York Academy of Sciences*, August 2009.

p. 196, regarding the link between meditation and the reduced activity of aging, inflammatory genes: "Yogic meditation reverses the NF-kB and IRF-related transcriptome dynamics in leukocytes of family dementia caregivers in a randomized controlled trial," *Psychoneuroendocrinology*, March 2013.

p. 196, regarding the link between fruit and vegetable portions and happiness and mental health: "Is psychological well-being linked to the consumption of fruit and vegetables?" *Social Indicators Research*, October 2012.

p. 196, regarding the link between processed foods and a higher risk of depression: "Dietary pattern and depressive symptoms in middle age," *British Journal of Psychiatry*, December 2009.

p. 197, regarding the link between exercise and psoriasis: "The association between physical activity and the risk of incident psoriasis," *Archives of Dermatology*, August 2012.

p. 198, regarding evidence that more exercise is not necessarily better: "Body fat loss and compensatory mechanisms in response to different doses of aerobic exercise—a randomized controlled trial in overweight sedentary males," *American Journal of Physiology*, September 2012.

p. 198, regarding evidence that working out twice per week boosts energy and fitness comparable to working out four and five times per week: "Combined aerobic/strength training and energy expenditure in older women," *Medicine and Science in Sports and Exercise*, January 2013.

INDEX